HOW TO GET A

Other titles in this series:

Bad Behaviour, Tantrums and Tempers
Confident Children
Good Habits, Bad Habits
Growth and Development
How to Teach your Baby to Sleep through the Night
The Secret of Happy Children
Starting School
Successful Potty Training
You Can Teach your Child to Read
You Can Teach your Child about Numbers

By the same author:

Successful Potty Training

Heather Welford

HOW TO GET A GOOD NIGHT'S SLEEP

A practical guide for parents of
wakeful babies and children

Thorsons
An Imprint of HarperCollinsPublishers

Thorsons
An Imprint of HarperCollins*Publishers*
77–85 Fulham Palace Road
Hammersmith, London W6 8JB
1160 Battery Street
San Francisco, California 94111–1213

Published by Thorsons 1995
10 9 8 7 6 5 4 3 2 1

© Heather Welford 1995

Heather Welford asserts the moral right to
be identified as the author of this work

A catalogue record for this book
is available from the British Library

ISBN 0 7225 3110 9

Printed in Great Britain by
HarperCollinsManufacturing Glasgow

All rights reserved. No part of this publication may be
reproduced, stored in a retrieval system, or transmitted,
in any form or by any means, electronic, mechanical,
photocopying, recording or otherwise, without the prior
permission of the publishers.

Contents

Acknowledgements		*vii*
Introduction		*ix*
Chapter 1	How Much – and How Often – Will My Baby Sleep?	1
Chapter 2	Your Newborn Baby – The First Three Months	8
Chapter 3	Older Babies	21
Chapter 4	Toddlers and Pre-schoolers	34
Chapter 5	Night-time and Its Terrors…	52
Chapter 6	Getting Help	59
Chapter 7	'It Worked for Me…'	71
Chapter 8	Questions	79
Useful Addresses		93
Index		94

Acknowledgements

I first heard about sleep problems back in the 1970s, when I joined the staff of *Parents* magazine. I soon realized that one of the major concerns our readers had – and which they wrote to us about – was sleep. Any feature about sleep always brought in a great response.

It's still the same. I am still answering readers' letters for the magazine, and mothers and fathers still ask us what to do about their baby, toddler or child who 'won't sleep'. More properly they mean 'won't sleep when we want him to' or 'keeps waking up'... and they can feel driven to distraction by the situation.

These parents have helped me write this book by sharing their experiences with me. My thanks to them and to the parents I have met through the National Childbirth Trust (especially the Newcastle branch, who were very welcoming to me when I visited some of their coffee mornings to quiz parents about their children's sleep in the course of my research).

Thanks, too, to health visitor Glenda Brown and her clients, who allowed me to sit in on Glenda's sleep clinic, and to consultant psychotherapist Dilys Daws, whom I have spoken to on a number of occasions about babies and sleep, and who has many sympathetic insights into the way families work and how babies behave.

Introduction

'When I ask parents about their new baby,' said a colleague, 'I never pose the question "Is he sleeping through the night yet?" Instead, I say something like "Is he getting you up much at night?" It seems so much gentler, somehow...'

I agreed. In fact, her reasoning for this small but important change was sound.

She recognizes that it is normal for babies to wake up at night. She knows from her own experience that the pressure is on parents for babies to 'sleep through' and, more specifically, for parents to somehow 'make' the baby 'sleep through'.

Parents, and especially mothers (and even more especially if they are breastfeeding) say they feel inadequate, even guilty, if their baby is waking up a lot at night. My friend's question neatly sidesteps this, and instead shows implicit support, and not criticism, if nights are hard to deal with.

For make no mistake: There's waking – and there's waking.

Dealing with a small baby who needs a quick feed or a cuddle once or even twice in the night and then goes back to sleep (with a small contented smile on his lips, even!), not to disturb you again until a civilized hour in the morning, is one thing. It's a thing, in fact, which most parents can learn to cope with, for a short time at least, as long as they are not made to feel that either they or their new baby is out of line in some way.

On the other hand, a crying, restless, fidgety, fussy, unhappy, screaming, tantrum-throwing, angry, frustrated baby or toddler or pre-school child who is like this once, twice, thrice or more every night as a routine is – to say the least – a little more difficult to bear.

Not all 'sleep problems' are the same – and the crying, restless, fidgety scenario is only one of the situations you will meet in this book, if not in your life as a parent. Other difficulties involve settling problems – when the process of going to bed in the first place is resisted, or delayed, or complicated by several attempts before success – as well as night-time fears, and early wakings.

We naturally associate sleeping difficulties of any sort with distress. We worry that a baby or toddler who wakes and cries in the night may be in pain, or even acutely anxious about something. These are, of course, very possible reasons for wakefulness at any age, young or old. This book will help you decide if your child is waking up because of these reasons, and will offer suggestions on what to do if he is. Just as important it will also attempt to give you guidance on what to do when there is basically nothing 'wrong' – except the wakefulness itself and the problems that result from it for you and the rest of your family.

This book will acknowledge that, sometimes, parents need help from outside. Being very close to a sleep problem, and suffering from consequent lack of sleep yourself, can mean you need support and a fresh pair of eyes on the issue.

This is much easier for us all to accept now, of course. Eighteen years ago, when I first began writing about family issues and first started hearing from parents of young children who wrote to *Parents* magazine, it was common for mothers and fathers to be told that their child's sleep problem was no more than a disciplinary matter – a simple example of 'bad behaviour'. The alternative view was that the situation demanded some pharmacological first-aid – that a bit of heavy doping could somehow literally knock the problem out ...

Fortunately, today's professionals concerned with the health of children and families are showing a real interest in sleep and

Introduction

in how they can help when sleep has become a problem. There is more good research and less folksy 'wisdom' masquerading as professional knowledge (and less implicit criticism of parents seeking help).

Understanding sleep and what happens when it goes 'wrong' in babies and children is something we don't need to leave to the professionals, however. We can inform ourselves, too; as a result we can be better parents, with babies and children we actually enjoy having around, and happier people – with a guarantee of a peaceful night's sleep (almost) every night!

1
· · · · ·

How Much – and How Often – Will My Baby Sleep?

Your baby may never sleep as much, or as often, as other babies you meet. Normal sleep needs differ from child to child and as a child grows – and there is a wide range in what is considered normal.

Babies typically change their sleep needs as they grow, and a five-year-old child is likely to sleep less than a newborn – but there may be a lot of ups and downs along the way. This book will help you and your baby adapt your needs for sleep – and for comfort and reassurance – to each other.

Published accounts of sleep needs describe the 'average' baby – don't forget there will be, by definition, many babies who need more, or less, sleep than the average.

One account describes a healthy newborn as sleeping about 16 or 17 hours in 24, in about seven sleep periods throughout the day and night.[1] By the age of three to four months, sleep needs have reduced to about 15 hours, in four or five periods. In a baby of this age, most of this sleep occurs at night. At six months the night-time sleep has stretched to 12 hours with occasional, brief wakings, and there will be in addition a couple of short naps of one or two hours' duration during the day.

Over the next year sleep changes again, mainly by the way the two daytime naps combine into one. In toddlerhood the nap is dropped at about the age of three, until at the age of five the 'average child' is sleeping for about 11 hours in every 24.

It can't be said too often – babies and toddlers and older

children who sleep a lot less than this average don't necessarily pose a problem. Indeed, even average children have the occasional non-average day, or days, or weeks. A change of surroundings or routine, or a slight illness, can all alter the sleep pattern.

In fact, it is probably more worrying, overall, if a baby sleeps for much longer than is typical. This can indicate illness or even an underlying developmental problem. This is unlikely to be the case if your baby has no other symptoms, however.

Sleeplessness in children may be compounded by settling problems and what has been termed 'sleep disruptions'[2] – and the two often go hand in hand. Settling problems can be defined as difficulty in getting the baby off to sleep in the first place, and sleep disruptions are those episodes in which sleep is broken and the child needs help in getting back to sleep – in settling – or else becomes increasingly more distressed.

It's safe to say that almost all parents experience both phenomena at some stage. It's a problem, though, if either of these situations begins to become a nightly routine, interfering with your own sleep to the extent that you try to influence your child's waking and settling ... and maybe you read a book like this in order to gain ideas and inspiration.

Don't feel that sleep problems are something you have to live with. Part of the difficulty you may face as a parent of a sleepless child is the guilt you feel at having the problem in the first place. This is made worse by feeling you 'ought' to do something about it – when you feel it is all your fault in the first place, how can you try to change your child? But sleeping patterns can change; you can take control; you are not a bad parent in wanting to do so.

Nine-month-old Christie's father worked away from home in the week. Her mother worked as a care assistant in an old people's home three nights a week. On these nights her grandmother had Christie to stay overnight at her house.

How Much – and How Often – Will My Baby Sleep?

Christie woke three our four times every night and was very difficult to settle back to sleep. This happened at her grandmother's house as well as at her own. She needed a bottle of warmed milk plus a lot of rocking, cuddling and reassuring each time before she fell back to sleep, exhausted with wriggling and crying.

Christie's mother, Jan, felt at a complete loss. She already felt guilty about working at all – she had always looked forward to staying at home with her baby, and this was why she only agreed to work nights when it became obvious the family needed the extra income. The days after she was at work she was tired, and the nights she slept at home were broken because of Christie's crying – and that made Jan feel worse. 'I can't be a proper mother, as I'm so tired. I sometimes resent Christie's demands – and that makes me feel worse.'

The family felt Christie was likely to be confused, sometimes waking up in Granny's house, sometimes in her own, sometimes with Daddy there, sometimes not. This had led them to accept disrupted sleep as a normal response on Christie's part, and meant they felt powerless to change the situation except by the drastic measure of either Jan or her husband giving up their job – something that was just not possible for practical and financial reasons.

Before any real attempt could be made to change Christie's pattern of sleeping and waking, Jan and Jan's husband and mother all needed to work through these feelings and accept that everyone would be better off if Christie could be helped to sleep better at night.

Jennifer sought help for her daughter's sleeping problem when Madeleine was 18 months old. Jennifer had tried to teach her to sleep through the night by leaving her to cry. This had meant three hours of hearing Madeleine scream, continuously and piteously. Jennifer felt like a bad mother, both for letting Madeleine cry and for (as she saw it) having a baby who wouldn't sleep. The crunch came when she saw her husband bury his head in his hands and weep as he heard Madeleine's distress.

Colin and Georgina felt their marriage was threatened by Joseph's crying. Neither could agree on how to manage the situation; each blamed the other at times, one for being soft, the other for being hard. Their tiredness meant they were irritable at work and at home. Someone told them their bad temper was causing Joseph's wakefulness and misery. This made them feel even worse.

One of the attendant difficulties with a sleep problem is that everyone has a theory about it, or an experience to share. Your next door neighbour, your auntie Mary, your childless friends even give their amateur two penn'orth when asked, and often when not. The professionals have their own ideas, too – the doctor, health visitor, midwife, nursery teacher and playgroup leader can throw in their opinions about what's causing it, and what you could do to cure it.

You can of course listen to their ideas and suggestions. They may help. But too often they only serve to make you feel criticized, resentful and confused. In particular, interventions from people close to you can be tricky. Grandparents may have strong ideas on how children should be brought up, and try to help by drawing on their own experiences. If you feel their approach is not right for you, it's almost the same as criticizing their parenting skills ... a sensitive area even a generation on.

This isn't to say you shouldn't seek help and support while going through your problem. This help can be professional or 'amateur', from friends you like and trust; if the help you get only serves to make you feel worse about the situation, or makes you feel undermined or criticized in any way, then ignore it! Most solutions or coping strategies only work when the person putting them into operation – i.e. you – believes in what he or she is doing.

DO YOU WANT TO CHANGE THE SITUATION?

Ask yourself if you are prepared to put up with your baby's crying, wakefulness, settling problems, fussing or whatever the situation is, rather than try to alter it.

Working out ways of coping, and waiting for change to happen by itself — as it sometimes does — is a perfectly acceptable alternative to actively working towards change.

Simply accepting that this is what your child is like at present, that these are her needs, and that you are there as a parent to meet them as far as you can, can lighten the load. The nightly battles and mutually contradictory needs (hers for company, yours for sleep, for example) which cause resentment and frustration, even in quite tiny babies, can ease ... making life easier to bear for everyone. Acceptance can improve your feelings about yourself as a parent, raising your confidence — and that can only be good for you and the people around you.

On the other hand, there is nothing wrong with deciding to change ... if you have realistic aims. There's no point, as we'll see, in trying to get a very new baby to sleep through the night without feeding. You are unlikely to get a wakeful, energetic toddler used to going to bed at 10 p.m. or later to feel happy and co-operative about a 6 p.m. bedtime.

Deciding on what would be acceptable and beneficial to you and your child and working towards it, and finding it works, is another way to boost your self-esteem and improve your relationships with your baby and the other members of your family. Read through parts of this book appropriate to you and your baby and then decide, if you are still unsure of what you feel or uncertain about what is right for you.

Get People on your Side

Whatever you decide to do, make sure all those involved in the care of your baby support you and are prepared to share in the decision. Sleep problems can be exacerbated by differences of approach and feeling between mother and father, for example. The effects of a sleep problem are undoubtedly made worse if one partner blames the other for causing it, or for not tackling it. Sometimes you may need to clear the air – perhaps with outside help – before deciding on how, or if, to tackle your baby's habits.

Jill:

Can you tell me whether or not I'm doing the right thing in going to my baby at night? She's 10 months old, and wakes up once or twice. She settles back to sleep with a breastfeed of a few minutes in length. My husband says I should stop feeding her, and just ignore her. He says I'm too soft. But I would hate to leave her to cry. I'd feel hard and even cruel.

Pauline:

I am trying to encourage my three-year-old son to feel it's bedtime at around seven o'clock – left to himself he would never admit he was tired, and he would keep going until he dropped. But when my husband works late he winds Tom up when he comes in. Tom is always excited to see his dad, and they have about half an hour of fun fighting and wrestling. It is always hard for Tom to calm down, and bedtime is a battle. My husband says he doesn't want Tom to be in bed when he comes home – that they both need to see each other, and in any case Tom's still in bed when my husband leaves for work in the mornings.

In both these situations both parents need to take time to work out a compromise – something that suits everyone's needs, including the child's. It could well be that these waking and settling problems throw up other differences in parenting styles that are, or will be in time, evident in other areas of these families' lives.

These need not be serious areas of conflict, of course. Most families can cope with a bit of inconsistency. However, these differences show up in the bedtime and waking difficulties, which happen several times a week, if not every night, and cause persistent irritation. It's worth tackling the situation ... in some way.

Jill, for instance, might want to think about talking over a time limit with her husband. She may feel her daughter still needs the comfort of night-time feeds – but be able to envisage a time when she could accept she won't. Alternatively, she may feel strongly enough to insist that as she is the one getting up and being disturbed, she can decide when and if to stop. It may be up to both partners to decide how big an issue this is to each of them, and to their daughter.

In Pauline's case, the time for Tom's dad to play with his son and to have that all-important contact he feels is necessary to the two of them is not just before bedtime. Or if it is, it could be calm, restful contact that Pauline can incorporate into the usual routine. Perhaps Tom's dad can read a story while Tom is already in bed. It could also help to work out a regular time when Tom and his dad can be together by arrangement – maybe a half-hour's or hour's football game at weekends, or a visit somewhere – something that's a more or less permanent fixture in the diary.

There will be more suggestions of ways through these situations at other points in this book.

ENDNOTES

1. Rebecca Huntley, *The Sleep Book for Tired Parents* (Souvenir Press, 1991).
2. Jo Douglas and Naomi Richman, *My Child Won't Sleep* (Penguin, 1984).

2

Your Newborn Baby – The First Three Months

It's always a bit arbitrary, setting a time when your baby stops being 'new'. But I've chosen the fairly conventional cut-off point of three months. This is approximately the length of time it seems to take for most babies and parents to become used to each other, and for the novelty on both sides to start becoming more of a routine.

Plenty of 'unsettled' babies (and we'll see soon who those are) take longer than three months to become calmer and easier to care for – conversely, some babies are sunny-tempered, placid and predictable long before this.

Even so, by three months (generally speaking) babies are more sociable and parents are more confident ... and beginning to make demands on life again, without being totally dominated by the needs of their baby. I say this from observation of the way families operate. The three-month mark has no real scientific basis as there is a wide range of 'normal', but crying, sleeplessness, restlessness and general unpredictability (and they often all go together) frequently show signs of improvement at around three months. I have known some babies who really lost their colicky behaviour at almost exactly three months, too (colic is sometimes even known as 'three-month colic', so this experience can't be all that unusual).

Your Newborn Baby – The First Three Months

LACK OF SLEEP – AND CRYING

Your baby has no other way of telling you something is wrong, other than by crying.

I can never agree with the sentiments of people who say things like 'that baby is only crying to get attention.' *Only* attention? Attention – someone to put the world right, someone to reassure them, someone to show they're not alone and needn't be frightened – is vital, and an essential part of survival. Leave babies without attention and they cannot live. And babies who are starved of love and affection – forms of attention, after all – may stay alive, but they don't thrive, in any physical or emotional sense.

Moreover, I don't buy the idea that a baby – and remember we are talking about a new and tiny person here, who understands very little indeed about the world – can work out ways of winding you up or manipulating you. I once heard a mother complain to another that her eight-week old baby had recently changed her sleeping habits and was starting to scream and scream at 3 a.m., after a couple of weeks of quite settled nights. 'I think they do it out of spite,' said the other mother. 'I'm quite sure of it.' I wanted to leap up and get her to explain herself – but I didn't. I think that idea is extraordinary: how can a little baby work out a plan and put it into action in this way?

Yet it's an indication of how helpless parents can feel in the face of new responsibility. Not only do we have to take charge of the physical care of this vulnerable little creature, we have somehow to keep it happy and socialized, too. It's hard, and sometimes overwhelming.

So it can be easy to believe babies can be manipulative when your resistance and your confidence are low. One part of you might be telling you how unsophisticated your baby is; another part might be telling you your screaming, unsettled and inconsolable baby is doing it to get back at you in some way, or out of some selfish idea that you don't deserve any sleep.

You may need support to help you see the situation in perspective. Accept all offers of help with household jobs. Say yes to babysitting or an offer to just sit with you and be an alternative pair of arms for your baby.

Sarah:

> *Esther cried and cried for the first 12 weeks of her life. I know she must have slept some of the time, but I could never really relax and appreciate the fact that she was sleeping and presumably content. I was always waiting for her to wake up again and start crying. I can remember longing for my husband's key in the door. When he came back from work I'd push a screaming Esther into his arms ... sometimes I was crying myself. Occasionally he'd manage to take a day off. Just having him at home then and at weekends made it easier to cope with.*

Let's look at ways a crying baby can be soothed to sleep.

- Sucking – at the breast, on a bottle, on a dummy.
- Rocking – in your arms, in a cradle, in a pram or pushchair.
- Cuddling.
- Wrapping – but don't wrap your baby up too tight or he could overheat. A thin sheet around him to keep his limbs still is all you need.
- Massage – you can use oil to massage your baby's skin. Baby oil is fine, or use a plain carrier oil such as almond oil, plus a little wheatgerm oil if your baby's skin is dry. For techniques see one of the specialist books on the market.[1]
- Touch – gentle stroking across the face, hands, feet – experiment to see what your baby prefers.
- A trip in the car (many parents end up driving round the block several times in the middle of the night – that's fine as long as your baby is safely strapped in, of course, and you're awake and calm enough to drive).

- Music or singing, or even gentle whispering in the ear.
- Listening to a 'soother' tape. There are a number of these on sale in major record stores. Most recommend starting as soon as possible after birth to get the best effect. The sounds or music have been specially chosen to 'mean' something to babies – there are, for example, simulated womb sounds designed to appeal to a baby still getting used to the 'outside' world.
- Moving to a different room, one which is quieter or even more noisy.
- Having someone else hold him – there's no way to prove it, but anxiety and stress do pass between the crying baby and the person holding him. Mothers in particular quite naturally get upset when their babies cry and they can't seem to console them.
- A change of position – over the shoulder, across the lap, on his tummy in your arms, on his back.
- Lying him down next to a warm, loving body (in your bed, with you, perhaps).

You will no doubt add other tricks to this list. Some of them will work some of the time; some will only work for a few moments – and then the baby wakes up again, crying as hard as ever. But they're all worth trying.

Checklist for Signs of Physical Discomfort

- Is he cold? Is he (far more likely) hot? You can get a good idea of your baby's temperature by feeling his chest or the back of his neck. If it feels hot then he is probably uncomfortable. Unless you've been told differently by your doctor, midwife or health visitor (because your baby is weak, or small, or was very pre-term, for example) your baby won't need more than one more layer of clothing or bedding than you do to feel comfortable. So if you're in a

T-shirt, all he'll need is a vest and a babygro. He doesn't need a cardigan and a shawl on top of that.
- Does he need a nappy change? Most babies really aren't aware of being in a wet or dirty nappy (and today's super-efficient disposable nappies keep them dry, anyway), but if they have a sore bottom because of nappy rash or thrush to start with, then they may be very uncomfortable. It's worth changing your baby's nappy as he may be soothed by the handling and human contact. If you're using terry towelling nappies, then of course you need to check for the almost proverbial nappy pin sticking in his skin ... just in case.
- Is he suffering the after-effects of an uncomfortable birth experience? Normally, the bones of the baby's skull move in a way that moulds the head as it descends through the birth canal. However, there are some osteopaths who feel it's possible for babies to be born with a headache because something goes wrong with this process and the skull bones exert an uncomfortable pressure until put right with manipulation. I have heard some convincing accounts of the way osteopathy has indeed helped crying babies. Of course you will make sure you see a qualified osteopath with a special interest in this sort of problem. It may take several visits to put the problem right, if it's going to work (see page 68).

You may think of other environmental and 'bodily' factors that could be disturbing your baby.

Is it Hunger?

A full tummy and a peaceful period of sleep go together in small babies. If your baby fails to sleep between feeds, it's natural to wonder if he isn't eating enough to satisfy his appetite.

If your baby is bottle-fed, he may need more milk than the

'average' quantities given as guidelines on the formula milk tin. Alternatively, think whether your baby may need to feed little and often – this is especially likely as a possibility at first. Be guided by your baby and what he seems to be trying to tell you. You won't always get it right ... but you will get better and better at it.

If your baby is breastfed, there may be more points to consider. Breast milk supply depends on the body getting the right 'messages' from the baby. The more your baby feeds, the more milk you make. If you try to limit or regulate the time or the frequency your baby is on the breast, and you may run the risk of making too little milk – it is normal for breastfed babies to feed often and at unpredictable intervals at first. This is not a pattern that lasts, however. As babies get more adept at feeding, and mothers' bodies get more efficient at producing milk, feeds tend to space themselves out, and to last for a shorter time.

So let your baby feed as often and as long as he wants to. This is good for him, you, and your milk supply. When he comes off the first breast, apparently finished feeding, offer him the second side after a short breather. He may or may not take it. It doesn't matter.

But – and it is a big 'but' – if your baby is still unhappy and seems to settle to a sound sleep only rarely despite free access to the breast, then something isn't right. Many mothers feel their babies are unsatisfied at the breast despite the fact that they are feeding them on demand. It is often helpful to get your health visitor or other experienced person to check that your baby is well-positioned at the breast, if you feel this way. You and your helper need to check that your baby's mouth is wide open when he comes to your breast, and that you're holding him chest-to-chest. His tongue needs to be forward, pushing his lower lip outwards. When he sucks, his jaw and his tongue will 'work' the breast in a way that's quite different from the sucking action used by a baby getting milk through a bottle teat.

A well-positioned baby – it's called 'being latched on' –

stimulates the breast to produce more milk, and also stimulates the let-down reflex which makes available the calorie-rich hind milk stored deep inside the breast. This can't happen if the baby is only sucking on the end of the nipple.

Poor positioning also makes you sore, and it can cause the nipples to crack and bleed ... sheer misery for you. From your baby's point of view, poor positioning means longer feeds because it takes longer to fill up when the let-down reflex is not working, and a less satisfying feeling of fullness. In some cases it's thought that tummy pains in babies can be caused by too much fore milk in relation to hind milk – an imbalance made more likely if the baby is not stimulating the let-down reflex.

If you're sure the positioning is right, and you still feel your baby is often hungry, build up your milk supply by fitting in extra feeds and by making sure your baby has as much time at the breast as he would like. If you're keen to breastfeed, giving bottles will undermine your milk supply as they disturb the supply-and-demand process – they fill your baby up and make him less eager for the breast. The different sucking technique of the teat can also confuse some babies and make them frustrated at the breast.

If your problem fails to improve, even with help, and you feel your baby needs more than you can give, then you may need to 'top up' your breast milk with formula. This is actually necessary in only a small number of cases, however – it's estimated that 98 per cent of women can fully breastfeed, given the right help, information and encouragement.

> Margaret's baby Joshua was restless and unhappy. Margaret herself had sore nipples which she coped with by curling her toes and gritting her teeth at every feed. When Joshua was 10 days old, Margaret's health visitor watched him feed. She managed to help Margaret correct Joshua's latching on – mainly by not bringing Joshua to the breast until his mouth was wide open. Margaret had got into the habit of slotting her nipple into Joshua's mouth

when it was only a little way open, and Joshua was sucking it in like a straw. It took a couple of days of practice, but once things went well feeds were shorter, with a more definite end, and Joshua slept more contentedly afterwards.

He Seems So Unsettled...

All babies – well, almost all – have some periods in the early days when nothing seems to keep them happy for long.

It's not uncommon for a baby to seem to find it difficult to sleep at about two to three days old, or perhaps in the first night or two back home if he's been born in hospital.

Babies do tend to perk up after the first couple of days – sometimes quite happily and sometimes apparently miserably. This is normal, and coincides with the time mothers often find their milk 'comes in' – when the colostrum their breasts produce at first changes to mature breast milk. It's natural for babies to be hungrier as the days pass, and the way babies show their hunger is to cry. Get help with positioning (*see above*) to ensure a satisfying feed.

If your baby is restless and unsettled when you first come home, it could be because the change in temperature, smell and so on are making him feel disconcerted. Just as at any other time, give your baby whatever comfort he needs to keep him happy.

Some babies are unsettled for a lot longer than these essentially transient stages, however. Many things can disturb them and cause them to cry. Noises, getting dressed or undressed, bathing ... it can be very tiring to look after a baby like this, but it seems to help if you simply accept that this is what your baby is like at the moment, that it won't last, and that giving him reassurance can build up his confidence in the world. If he prefers quiet, don't take him to noisy places. If he hates a bath, top and tail him with warm water on your lap or lying down in front of you, instead.

It's very common for young babies to be unsettled in the evenings, whether they are breast- or bottle-fed. Some babies seem to work up to this from about the middle of the afternoon onwards. Don't try to fight this – it's tempting to try and put your baby in his cot or his pram as soon as you feel he may be asleep, but you can then find you get increasingly more cross as your evening's peace is disturbed again and again. Catnapping seems to be normal at this age, at this time of the day – babies grow out of this, and if they don't they can be helped to develop a more settled afternoon and evening when they're a little older (*see page 22*).

Bryony:

My daughter was very wakeful in the evenings from the age of about two weeks. She dropped off to sleep for no more than a few minutes at a time. She was on and off the breast for hours. Someone suggested I give her a bottle at about six o'clock to settle her down, and while it seemed to work the first couple of nights, it made no difference in the long term. She started to fight the bottle, and got herself even more cross and bad-tempered. In the end I just sat with her in my arms for most of the evening – I made the evening meal in the morning, so I wouldn't be so rushed later on, and forgot about other jobs ... it was the only way for us.

Wakeful Nights, Sleepy Days ...

Occasionally, a new baby gets his days and nights mixed up. That is, the longest sleep happens in the hours of daylight, when you're up and about, and the night-time is characterized by short naps and frequent feeds.

How or why this happens is unclear – and in any case, it doesn't really matter. You can decide to live with it, as it tends to resolve itself in a few weeks as your baby's body clock sorts itself out to follow the human animal's natural diurnal rhythm. Alternatively, some parents have found that waking the baby in the daytime, and offering more feeds, can gradually alter the pattern. If you decide to do this, keep night feeds very low key, in the dark as far as possible, and avoid nappy changes unless your baby has a sore bottom or the nappy has leaked.

Don't Blame Yourself

Mothers may be told their crying, wakeful baby is 'picking up your anxiety'. Crying babies cause anxiety, naturally enough, and if you're trying to cope with this anxiety on top of your own fatigue because of the lack of sleep – caused, again, by your baby's wakefulness – you're going to be even more stressed.

Babies are sensitive; they may well be less comfortable in the arms of someone who feels awkward and tense; they may cry as a result. But I don't believe they are mind-readers. Do everything you can to reduce the physical signs of your tension – relaxation exercises, a small alcoholic drink, music, watching a comedy show on TV. Share the cuddling and rocking and whatever else you need to do with someone else as often as you can. Put all unnecessary tasks such as ironing and cleaning on the non-urgent list.

Now, how on earth is your baby going to know you're anxious if you don't give him any clues? Just give him what he needs at the moment, accept that it won't last forever, and seek out non-critical support from the people around you.

Can Babies Be 'Spoiled' in this Way?

No.

Call me soft – but I am convinced a tiny baby's wants are the same as his needs. He hasn't the brain power or the experience to distinguish between his urgent need for comfort, milk, company or whatever, and your desire to teach him his place in the world. Meeting his needs teaches him he is loved, he matters, he's safe, you're there ... later, when he develops more of a memory and more understanding, the process of negotiating his wants can begin.

Is the Baby Ill?

Don't be afraid to ask your doctor's advice if you feel your baby may be genuinely ill or in pain. You may want to talk to the doctor on the phone instead of calling him or her out, outside surgery hours – though many worried parents are only truly reassured if the baby can be actually seen by a doctor. Ill babies tend not to cry and cry; they are more likely to be listless, sleepy, difficult to feed – if the only symptom your baby has is his constant crying, he is more than likely to be hale and healthy. All GPs experience the anxious middle-of-the-night, desperate phone call, with the baby screaming in the background. By the time the home visit actually takes place the baby is often sleeping peacefully ... one doctor told me 'Yes, it can be irritating, but I'd far rather make a visit and find the baby was fine, after all. I understand how worried parents can get.'

Colic

Colic is often used by health professionals and parents to explain the frequent, excessive bouts of crying suffered by small babies, usually under six months at the most. It's thought to keep babies awake, and to waken them up when they're asleep. It's not really an explanation, however, as no one has come up with a totally satisfactory cause of colic.

Definitions of what constitutes 'frequent' or 'excessive' crying vary in the literature, and I'm not going to add to the confusion by saying what I think is excessive or frequent. It becomes a problem when the carers of the baby feel overwhelmed and are frequently unable to comfort the baby when he cries –

Your Newborn Baby — The First Three Months

however long or short a time it has been according to the clock.

Colic is sometimes said to be the result of an immaturity in the digestive system. Drugs prescribed for colic are formulated to prevent spasms in the intestines, which are thought to cause pain.

There is very little evidence, however, to show that what goes on in the digestive system of a 'colicky' baby is any different to what goes on in a non-colicky baby's. Put your ear to the tummy of a peaceful sleeping baby and you'll hear all sorts of glugs and gurgles, which don't disturb the baby at all.

It could be, as Sheila Kitzinger suggests[2] (in my view quite plausibly) that digestion has something to do with it, because some babies are more distressed than others at the normal feelings associated with the workings of the digestive system. This distress is compounded when his mother becomes anxious at his wrigglings and writhings. This is an explanation that in the wrong hands could come perilously close to blaming the mother for 'causing' her baby's colic, of course, so it needs to be handled with care. That is far from what Kitzinger means, and it's worth reading her book for her mother-centred, sympathetic approach to the crying baby, whether or not you have been told your baby has colic.

Colic, as mentioned, is sometimes termed 'three-month colic'; whatever it is, it often does clear up by then.

Wind

Wind, like colic, is often posited as a reason for wakefulness and crying in a new baby.

Wind, or gas as the Americans call it, is as much of a dark mystery as colic. If a baby cries, someone will suggest 'he has wind'... though why air, which is always present in the stomach, should sometimes cause pain is not clear. An air bubble might distend the stomach, perhaps — as adults we can feel uncomfortable, even pained, by trapped gas in the intestines or stomach, and it's worth wondering if the same phenomenon affects babies.

Some babies do seem to be calmed once they've burped after a feed, though the consensus among experts used to handling babies is that there is no need to help the burp on its way by a lot of back-rubbing or patting. Merely sit the baby up so that any air has a straight route up towards the mouth.

It could be worth giving a wakeful, crying baby the chance to burp after a feed – if you think it works, then carry on doing it. It cannot do any harm at all.

I am unconvinced that wind can regularly wake a baby up, however – babies burp (and even fart, for that matter) loudly if they need to, unrestrained by any notions of politeness. But plenty of mothers disagree with me. The jury is still be out on this one, though I'd like to knock on the head the very common idea that babies have a thin blue line above the upper lip when they 'have wind'. Look closely and you will see that most white babies have the sort of translucent skin that allows tiny veins to show up as blue. Why on earth would these veins show up more on the lip because of gas in the stomach?

ENDNOTES
1. Margaret Fawcett, *Aromatherapy for Pregnancy and Childbirth* (Element Books, 1992). The author does not recommend the use of essential oils for very young babies.
2. Sheila Kitzinger, *The Crying Baby* (Viking, 1990).

3

Older Babies

If your baby is three months old or so and still waking regularly, you aren't doing anything wrong – and neither is she.

This is also true of the baby who is still without a regular bedtime which gives you and your partner or any other older people in the household a 'free' evening.

However, now's the time to consider certain changes to your baby's lifestyle if you would like a more predictable and more peaceful evening and night.

Looking at settling in the evening first, think about working towards a routine each night. One fairly typical and easy-to-operate sequence of events is suitable for babies from around three months of age – and works with older babies than this, too.

The idea behind it is to teach your baby about bedtimes, and about how the pace and routine of the family (as far as she's concerned, anyway) accommodate this regular feature. By now, your baby has probably developed an appreciation of basic truths – such as the fact that there are special people in her life who love and care for her, that she can recognize them and that they recognize her. They have the same face and voice every time she sees them. She knows at some level that the cot or pram or wherever she sleeps are 'hers' – though of course she still doesn't know or care about possessions and possessiveness. These places are familiar to her. She may be a baby who resists going into the sleeping place awake, as she knows she is likely to

How to Get a Good Night's Sleep

be left there alone, or at least away from the cuddles and hugs she thrives on.

(Many babies, in fact, have not yet learned to fall asleep by themselves at this age, and they may have stayed with the newborn pattern of dropping into a deep contented sleep on the breast or the bottle. This is all right for the moment and need not pose a problem – but when your baby gets older it may need changing (*see page 22*).

You can capitalize on your baby's memory and experience when you try to establish a regular evening routine.

Here's a couple of real-life examples of families who decided now was the time to change.

Helena's daughter Katherine was 14 weeks old and going to bed for her longest sleep at about 9 or 9.30 every night. She quite often had a short early evening nap of about an hour or so, at about 5.30 or 6 o'clock. She was still fully breastfed.

Helena was quite happy to continue breastfeeding Katherine, and to give her a last breastfeed in the evening – but the last breastfeed after 9 o'clock was ceasing to be convenient. She decided it would be useful for Katherine to go to bed at about 7 o'clock. This would mean Helena could start attending an evening class she was interested in and which began at 7.30.

Ruth's son Thomas was nine months old and used to late nights and late mornings. He slept through the night and had done so since the age of about five months – but didn't go to bed until about 10.30, waking up to start the day well after 9 o'clock on most mornings. That used to suit Ruth and her husband Bob – whoever was around at night gave Thomas his night-time bottle, and he was happy to take it from either Ruth, Bob or Ruth's mother, who occasionally babysat. The late mornings meant Ruth could get on with some household jobs before Thomas needed to be got up and given breakfast. But Thomas was starting to be irritable in the evenings, and the family thought he would benefit

Older Babies

from earlier nights. However, Ruth didn't fancy the idea of Thomas waking up at 6 instead of 9 ... she needed to work out a way of settling him earlier without paying the price of an unacceptably early morning.

The basic formula of an evening routine is quite simple: the same things are done in the same order each night. What these things are and the order in which and what time you actually do them are less important factors than the actual establishment of a consistent nightly regime.

The atmosphere of your house is crucial, too. If you have a very busy family life, with older children and their friends making a lot of noise, eating at different times, and coming and going all the time, then your baby's bedtime preparations are going to suffer. Older babies don't care to miss out on any action that's going – and they can easily get wound up when there's a great frenzy of people and activity.

Try to encourage people to calm down in the evening or, if that's not possible, remove your baby from the centre of things some time before you actually expect her to fall asleep.

Think about what you already do, or could do with your baby to make the evening a pleasant, companionable and quiet time. You might give her a breast- or bottle-feed; give her a bath; give her a snack or a meal; look at a book together; sing some songs to her; snuggle up with her and cuddle her; chat with her about the day's happenings. A suggested routine for a six-month-old baby on solids plus breastmilk might look like this:

4.00 p.m.: snack – short breastfeed plus piece of fruit.
5.30 p.m.: tea; milk from a cup with a lid (the breastfeed might send her to sleep before you want her to).
6.00 p.m.: bathtime.
6.15 p.m.: last breastfeed.
7.00 p.m.: into the cot.

A routine for a rather older baby could be like this:

- 4.00 p.m.: snack, play session with older sibling in from school.
- 5.00 p.m.: tea with sibling and others who are around.
- 6.00 p.m.: story time or a quiet look through books together, away from busier parts of the house.
- 6.30 p.m.: bathtime.
- 7.00 p.m.: last breast or bottle feed.
- 7.30 p.m.: into the cot.

CHANGING YOUR BABY'S PATTERN

It might take a while to establish a pattern in such a way that your baby comes to expect the same order of activities. If your baby is used to having a nap in the evening – perhaps she drops off into a doze at any time from mid-afternoon onwards – you may have to think of ways to prevent her from doing this. The younger your baby is, the more difficult it is to distract her into wakefulness. If she needs to sleep, she may well do so no matter what you do – and be irritable and fractious if you try to prevent her.

You can, however, influence your baby's sleeping and waking by trial and error. For example, if your baby habitually falls asleep in the back of the car at around 3.30 when you drive back from the shops or from collecting other children from school, perhaps she may be asleep for a couple of hours – especially if she hasn't had a longish nap earlier in the day. You may have developed a routine of carrying her out of the car and placing her carefully somewhere she can continue her sleep until she wakes up. This, though, makes it hard to expect her to be ready for a long sleep not two hours later – she's more likely to awaken refreshed and raring to go. So, see what happens if you gently waken her as soon as you get home, or after a much shorter time than usual.

Make sure anyone who looks after your baby in the evening sticks more or less to the same routine, even when you're not there. You may have problems when you go on holiday, or if you are on a long journey away from home – but try as far as you can to stay with the sequence of events (*see more on holidays, page 2*).

Changing the Daytime Routine

Many babies quite naturally have a longish sleep in the morning plus a further nap or two before the night comes.

Left to themselves, babies are likely to cut out one or two naps at some time during the first year – and there are some who rarely sleep in the day, grabbing no more than the occasional catnap if they happen to be in a buggy or the back of a car when they are tired.

Think about when it would suit you to have your baby asleep for a predictable, regular time. You may be able to combine two existing naps into one.

> Jennifer's daughter Rose is seven months old. She still breastfeeds and is also on three good solid meals a day. She wakes at about 7 each morning and has her breakfast at about 7.30. By 10 o'clock or 10.30 she's already flagging and needs to sleep somehow – Jennifer manages to put her in her cot most days, but on other days they are not in the house at that time and Rose falls asleep in the car or the pram, or even on Jennifer's lap if they're visiting at someone else's house. She sleeps until lunchtime, especially if she's in her cot and left undisturbed. By 5 o'clock she is sleepy again, and often has another hour or so. Bedtime at the moment is 8.30 or 9 p.m. Jennifer feels that it would suit her better to have Rose asleep after lunch so she's tired again by the evening – though she doesn't see that Rose could do without her morning nap just yet.

Jennifer's situation could be changed, or at any rate Jennifer could try to change it by making Rose's morning nap as short as possible. She could then try putting Rose down to sleep after lunch – it could be that Rose is tired enough by then to feel happy to sleep. The advantage of this is that one single nap in the middle of the day leaves the possibility open that Rose will be ready for bed rather earlier in the evening. Jennifer could combine this change with an evening teatime-bathtime-breastfeed routine. In time Rose may well manage to skip her morning nap, though there may be a period when she falls asleep exhausted in the late morning – before she has had her lunch. Jennifer will do well during this time to bring Rose's lunch forward to make the most of the 'full tummy' effect so Rose really does sleep as long as she needs to.

Early Risers

It's probably true to say that the majority of babies go through at least some stage when they wake up earlier than you – and seem reluctant to go back to sleep until a more civilized hour. Newer babies can often be fed back to sleep; older babies won't be fooled. It's morning for them, and action time...

At the moment, Henry, who's 10 months, wakes up at about 5.30 – and starts shouting and yelling for us. He can pull himself up to standing in his cot, and since he's learned to do that it seems to make him even more determined to start the day.

Emma is 14 months. She wakes up in the mornings at 6.30, which is much too early for us, winter or summer. At first I used to bring her into bed with us and snuggle up with her. This doesn't calm her down for long. She wants us to play with her. She's begun trying to prise our eyelids open with her fingers when she sees us lying there, eyes shut in a pretence of sleep.

Older Babies

Here are some of the tricks you might try to keep your early riser from needing your attention too soon:

- Check that her bedroom curtains don't let in too much light.
- Make sure her room is neither too cold nor too hot in the early morning.
- Leave some safe toys in her cot, the sort she can play with without coming to any harm.
- Make her room interesting to look at, with mobiles and pictures.
- Leave a drink within reach (water is the safest for her teeth).
- Check there is no morning noise rousing her to action – is her cot against a wall where she can hear your neighbour coming in from night shift …?

If and when these measures fail, here's how to make it easier for you to cope:

- Give in, get up, give her breakfast and listen to the farming programme on the radio.
- Bring her into your room, shut the door if she's mobile, and have a few toys on the floor you can help her play with without you needing to get out of bed.
- Give her a breast- or bottle-feed in your bed – it might just soothe her enough for you to grab a little more relaxation, if not sleep.

Above all, remember that this stage does not last a long time – it seems in many cases to be a genuine physical response to a stage of sleep development. With children under about 15 months, early waking seems associated with a real energy and commitment to starting the day – and you cannot make a baby as lively and as wakeful as this go back to sleep, or expect her to amuse herself for very long without needing your attention.

Night Waking

Despite what you may hear and what other people tell you your baby ought to be doing, once she gets beyond the newborn stage it is normal for babies to continue waking at night, needing attention and showing distress when they don't get it.

Not all mothers and fathers think this is too much of a problem.

Mandy:

> *Everyone I meet asks me if Josh is still waking up. He is eight months, and if I say I haven't had a full night's sleep since he was born it sounds very dramatic. It's true, though. He usually gets back to sleep OK once I pop his dummy back in. I can do it in my sleep, almost, and at the moment it doesn't really bother me. I wouldn't like to think I was still getting up to him in six months' time, though.*

Yvonne:

> *Peter sleeps with us. He wriggles and wakes several times a night. He is nearly a year, and getting bigger all the time, so when he moves about it does wake me more than it used to. But I seem to be able to survive on broken nights — I'm the sort of person who can get back to sleep again fairly quickly, fortunately.*

For other parents, it's a source of stress.

Older Babies

Jayne:

All my friends with babies say Laura should be going through the night, now she's seven months and on three solid meals a day. I wish she would as well. She needs a lot of settling to get her to sleep in the first place, and when she wakes up we have to go through the whole process of bottle, rocking, bottle, rocking, to get her to go back down again. It can take an hour or so each time. I wish there was some way I could make sure she slept through until morning. I find I'm irritable and touchy most days, and I feel sure lack of sleep is making me feel this way.

Ben:

Please tell us how we can get our son to stay asleep. At the moment my wife feeds him every time he wakes, but this seems to be becoming more frequent, especially as he has fewer breastfeeds in the day than he used to. He wakes up four, sometimes five times a night, and I would have thought that at 11 months old he should be getting the food and drink he needs in the day. I wake up every time he does, though my wife tries to get to him before he cries loudly enough to wake me. I have tried to settle him down, to wean him off the breast in the hope he won't wake up, but he just screams and screams. Neither of us would be happy to stop him breastfeeding, as he seems to need it so much.

One useful, recently published study threw some welcome light on what older babies actually do.[1] Out of the 15,000 parents surveyed, 640 had babies of about six months of age.

The first question asked was 'How many hours does your baby sleep at night?' Answers ranged from one hour to 15 hours, with the mode being 12 hours (the mode is the most commonly occurring number – more of these babies, therefore, slept for 12 hours than any other number of hours). Sixteen per cent of the babies – well over one in every 10 – had no regular sleeping pattern.

The parents were also asked if their babies slept through the night – that is, were those night-time sleep hours unbroken? Only 16 per cent regularly slept through. Fifty per cent woke occasionally. Five per cent woke once every night, and a further 17 per cent woke more than once every night (ranging from twice to eight times). Nine per cent woke up most nights. This means that a third or thereabouts of babies aged six months are waking up most nights or every night, with half of the ones that wake doing it more than once.

Interestingly, the study also asked what parents did in response to their baby's wakeful cries. The most popular response – chosen by 23 of cent of parents as something they 'always' did – was rocking or cuddling. A further 49 per cent of parents did this 'usually' or 'sometimes'. Next in popularity – the thing parents 'always' did – was to give the baby a dummy (*for more on dummies see page 79*), which tied in terms of numbers with giving the baby a drink of milk (presumably most likely a breast- or bottle-feed at this age, though some babies will have a cup by now). Only 51 per cent of parents 'never' brought their baby into bed with them, but only 8 per cent 'always' did. The remaining 41 per cent did this 'sometimes' or 'usually'. Other strategies included changing the nappy or giving a drink (other than milk).

Twenty-eight per cent of six-month-olds routinely sleep in the same room as their parents.

What does all this tell us? As the author of the published report points out, 'Knowing their baby's behaviour is "normal" and shared by many other babies of the same age is often reassuring to parents.'

Further surveys have shown us that a baby's sleeping patterns change throughout the first year anyway. The parents who worry that their wakeful baby will still be wakeful in six months' time may be worrying needlessly. Conversely, some babies who have slept well at first start to wake up, sometimes frequently.

Older Babies

It is hard to see how parents can influence these patterns, which can come and go bewilderingly. But there are things you can try — if your baby's wakefulness is interfering with your enjoyment of parenthood, if you are finding it hard to get back to sleep again, or if you feel your baby is genuinely unhappy at night and that this is making it hard for her to settle back to sleep after waking.

- Give your baby a chance to get back to sleep on her own, without going into her. I don't propose leaving her to cry it out, or to cry herself back to sleep — separation anxiety tends to start in the second half of the first year, and it's a very normal and natural response for your baby to want to be with you when you're not there. But a few minutes' whimpering may be all there is to it — and it could allow your baby to fall back to sleep without fully waking.
- Keep anything you do at night very low key. If your baby wakes before you have gone to bed yourself, don't bring her downstairs in front of the TV or the family. Keep feeds as short as you can and try not to play with or interact with your baby in a way that will rouse her even more.
- If you can make the sleep place in the day the same as the night, this helps your baby associate her cot with the same activity at all times.
- Encourage the use of a soft toy, blanket or special cloth at bedtime. You may have to take on board the risk of this becoming a part of your child for the next few years — but so what?
- You can start actively teaching your child to sleep through if you like (*see page 48*), although many professionals working with babies and children don't try this before the age of around a year. It can work with younger babies, though, and I have heard of parents doing it with babies of as young as four or five months.

- Accept that your baby is not likely to be hungry at this age – and that depriving her of a bottle or the breast in the middle of the night is not going to affect her nutritionally (note: this applies to healthy, thriving babies who are on solid food. If your baby has been ill or seriously underweight, see your doctor before you decide to drop any night feeding). This may help you feel strong enough to withhold this – but it is your choice. You may find you don't mind feeding in the night, especially as babies get such a lot of comfort and reassurance from the familiar.

WHAT COULD BE MAKING YOUR BABY WAKE AND NEED YOU?

Apart from the fact that she's still a baby, still learning about getting to sleep on her own, and her need for reassurance, of course ...

- Teething? The now-traditional doctor's dictum that 'teething causes nothing but teeth' grew up in response to the old and daft ideas that teething caused fatalities in susceptible infants. It's been left to mothers, on the whole, over the last 40 years or so to uphold the notion that babies whose teeth are coming through suffer pain and misery which may prevent them sleeping. But one study asked mothers to record symptoms noticed in their babies, and got them to note down when the first tooth erupted as well.[2] Surprisingly, perhaps, there *was* a connection between feverishness and the tooth coming through in a greater number of children than would be expected by chance. So, on this basis it could mean that some babies are prevented by their symptoms from a calm night's sleep. (Always see your doctor if you think your baby might be ill, of course. Don't just put it down to teething.)

- Nightmares? Sometimes mothers and fathers do feel their baby is actually frightened, perhaps by a bad dream. This is possible, though we cannot be sure when dreams start. Babies do show signs of fear before they can talk. It's probable that bad dreams are no more than an occasional cause of sleep difficulties in babies, however.
- Wind or colic? By now, doctors tend to dismiss the likelihood of wind or colic waking a baby and preventing her from settling again, and it does seem improbable that the digestive system should take this long to settle down, in the absence of any other signs of allergy or intolerance. But wind and colic have at best a shaky claim to being clinical conditions anyway, as we've seen (*pages 18–20*). I have heard from many mothers who are quite sure their babies of six, nine, 12, 15 months or more are suffering from wind, nevertheless — but I would still incline to the view that babies of this age, if they're healthy and thriving, are probably waking up for other reasons and just need help — if not now then later — in getting back to sleep by themselves.
- Change in surroundings? Yes, some babies find it hard to get back to sleep if they wake up, recognize they're somewhere strange (perhaps on holiday) and become bewildered. It can start a new pattern. In time your baby may settle back to the former pattern — if not, keep night-time reassurance brief and low key, and think about making more specific changes to the way you deal with it (*see page 48*).

ENDNOTES

1. The Avon Longitudinal Study of Pregnancy and Childhood is looking at many aspects of health and care of babies born in 1991 and 1992 in the Avon area. The results of the sleep survey of these families are published in *Professional Care of Mother and Child*, August/September 1994, Vol. 4, No. 6.
2. L. Jaber, I. J. Cohen, A. Mor, 'Fever associated with teeth', *Archives of Disease in Childhood* 1992; 67: 233–4.

4

Toddlers and Pre-schoolers

Once a baby grows into toddlerhood – over the age of, say 12–15 months – things change. Your baby is now more of a person with a separate and distinctive personality. He can walk, even run away from you or what you want him to do. He has language – first his understanding of your language starts to develop, and then of course he begins to express his own feelings, wants and preferences through speech which you and others can understand. He begins to comprehend with crystal clarity that sometimes you want one thing and he wants another. He also knows that sometimes he wants something and there is no way it is going to happen … he's physically unable to make it happen, or some stronger force than him (you?) is saying he can't.

This is often the underlying cause of many toddler frustrations and episodes of anger and rage – the sort of episodes we call 'tantrums' or symptomatic of 'the terrible twos'.

When it comes to sleep and settling, problems with waking or difficulties in settling in the first place can be compounded by tantrums. We also expect to be able to 'tell' our toddlers to go to sleep, and for this to work because we know they have language, actively and passively. After all, we reason, he knows the meaning of the words. He doesn't have the excuse, or the luxury, of not being able to understand what on earth we mean when we put him in a cot, turn off the light, say 'good night' and walk away!

Toddlers and Pre-schoolers

Trouble is, not sleeping is one of the ways children have of retaining their autonomy. This is a world which encourages independence, where doing things on your own is complimented – what a clever boy! You've eaten all your dinner with your spoon! – and it's also a stage where a child is 'programmed' to branch out into discovery and adventure, finding things out by himself and delighting in his increased physical and mental prowess. Not going to sleep is a great way of being your own person, of affecting the world and the other people in it who are close to you.

At the same time, this little person wants and needs your love, approval and affection, which are demonstrated by your company and attention – which he can never get enough of, on his terms.

It's no wonder that waking up, needing to be settled again, waking up, needing to be settled again ... is such a common scenario, night after night, in many families. When asked, 17 per cent of mothers of infants aged between one and two rated their children as having moderate or severe sleep problems.[1] A well-known and oft-quoted study of parents of three-year-olds showed that 14 per cent of children and their families were affected by sleep problems, a figure which rose to 27 per cent of those who had other behavioural difficulties.[2]

It's no accident, either, that the other common bones of contention between parents and their toddlers are eating and potty training. Many families have a series of mealtime struggles; they want their toddler to eat ... the toddler doesn't want to eat. Or the toddler eats, but only certain foods, prepared in a certain way. Or only at certain times – usually between normal mealtimes. 'You cannot make me eat,' the toddler seems to be saying, 'this is a power I grant to myself.' It's the same with potty training: bowel and bladder functioning can't be switched on and off according to the will of anyone but the owner of said bladder and bowel.

This isn't to imply that your child is figuring all this out in a way to manipulate you. Far from it. A toddler's night-time behaviour reflects his confusion and his conflicting needs and feelings, not any darker underside of his character. It's the same with eating and potty training. Also, these behaviours become learned and develop their own momentum. It becomes hard to unravel their effects and their causes.

With a sleep problem, there is also the fact that many toddlers have not yet learned, or have forgotten, how to get to sleep themselves. They wake up, they want to go back to sleep again (because they're tired) but can't because of this inability to do it just by 'telling' themselves or by shutting their eyes once more.

Being a parent of a toddler is a great mixture of highs and lows.

Jen:

Louis is two. He wakes up three or four times every night. He stands up in his cot, rattling the bars and whimpering. The whimpering gets to be screams in a short time. Sometimes he has his eyes almost shut, and his head is flopping — but he still yells. He needs me to go in, calm him down, cuddle him and then place him down in his cot again when he's dropped off to sleep in my arms. It takes about 10 minutes each time. Then he may wake up an hour or two later, in exactly the same state.

Amanda:

Charlotte is three. She used to be a good sleeper but in the last three months she has become difficult to settle. I think it started when we were on holiday and she had a slight fever. I didn't like to leave her on her own to get to sleep, so I stayed with her while she dropped off and went to her as soon as I heard her wake in case she felt poorly. When we got home she told me she wanted me to stay with her when she went to sleep, holding her hand. She hates me to leave or to drop her hand before she finally falls asleep. She is OK for the rest of the night, usually, anyway — but I would like to be able to let her go to sleep on her own. I've tried to explain that she's a big girl now and should be able to do so — but she just says 'Mummy, I really love you lots when you stay...'

Kim:

Night-times are just a part of the situation we're in with Tom. He's 28 months and he used to be such a lovely little boy, sociable and outgoing. He's still lovely, and we have a lot of fun — when things are going well. He seems to want to have his own way in everything. He only eats bread, crisps, apples and biscuits, and drinks milk and orange juice. That's it. Any attempts to get him to eat more or other things lead to a tantrum — we've tried absolutely everything and nothing works. I'm trying to potty train him as well, and I'm positive he's got the idea — he says things like 'Tom do wee in potty...' — but we can go through six pairs of wet pants in a morning. At night he just comes in with us when he wakes, and I wouldn't mind except he demands my attention at night and won't let me sleep. He wriggles and kicks, and sings, anything to engage me in some sort of conversation, even if it's just yelling at him to stop! Sometimes in the day he will just drop off into a deep sleep, say when he's playing on the floor with his cars, or the minute he gets into the pushchair if we have to go to the shops, so I suspect he's tired a lot of the time. I do get mad with him, partly because I'm tired myself, and then I feel guilty because I've lost my temper. I look at his little face and remind myself he's only a baby...how can he cope with my irritation and anger? I know it sounds a mess — I don't know where to begin to sort him, and me, out.

Kim's situation is typical of that of many parents who have written to me over the years — often at great length. You can hear the lack of confidence, the self-doubt and the mixed feelings in every sentence. Just when parenthood is starting to feel like something you might get good at, given enough practice, the whole notion that you've got it taped is challenged by a new set of dilemmas, compounded by the fact that you get so tired it's hard to see how you can work out a solution.

The best bit of advice you can follow, as a starting point, is to stop trying to do everything at once. Don't try to tackle each and every difficulty you have with your child at the same time – you will spend all day and night saying 'no', being negative, and leaving no room for negotiation, fun and enjoyment.

In Kim's case, it's simply not a good idea to tackle potty training at present. It will make no difference in the long term whether Tom uses the potty or loo now or in six months' time. When the situation becomes an issue of persuasion, or even discipline, you can set yourself up for a long haul – and ultimately your child can win this one, until he decides it's better for him to be trained. At present Tom has no real benefit to gain from compliance, except his mum's approval, which probably doesn't mean a lot at the moment. He's too young to be bothered by what anyone else thinks of him. Later he may appreciate the convenience of dry pants and no nappy, and feeling part of the 'big kid' community – most children under three (and often older) couldn't care less.

It's never worth your while to try to make your child eat more, or more varied foods, either. Gentle persuasion is fine; making mealtimes enjoyable so he'll want to join in is OK, too. But making the issue strongly related to approval, or making accusations of naughtiness if food isn't eaten, really can make the problem worse. Eating well is a social matter as well as a nutritional one – and it is a nuisance and a slight embarrassment, let's face it, when food is rejected in this firm, unyielding way. The point to remember is that healthy, well-loved children don't starve themselves, and that making a good diet available and attractive is all you can do. Many children, in fact, get what they need from an apparently very limited diet. Tom's list of likes isn't very long, but it's good, for example, that he drinks milk and fruit juice, and eats bread! Kim's health visitor could talk this over with Kim and work out whether Tom needs a vitamin and mineral supplement, just to ensure he doesn't go short of any important nutrients.

It may well be that tackling the sleep problem is a priority for many families, particularly if it's interfering with their own chance to sleep. When you're constantly tired, every other problem seems mountainous. As some parents suspect, their child is suffering from tiredness too, in some cases, and this makes it more likely that his temper will fray easily in the day as well.

Think about what is most important to you, and decide when and if you are going to deal with it now or later.

DOING NOTHING ...

You always have the option not to do anything, and to accept that this is the way things are at present. Making this decision can be a positive move in itself. It means you aren't constantly fighting with your child, nor with anyone else close to you who keeps throwing in useful (or otherwise) suggestions on what you can do.

Doing nothing about a sleep or settling problem – to get back specifically to the topic of this book – could mean you won't get as angry and as cross about the problem, whether or not you have shown these feelings to your child. It means that you will carry on doing whatever you have been doing, but with good grace. Do you get into bed with your child in the middle of the night? If so, do so and stay there instead of lying awake waiting for the first second you can nip back to your own bed before your child wakes – or without waking your child as you do it. Do you keep moaning at your child and bringing the subject up in front of him during the day – or even tackling him about it in the same way? Doing nothing will mean staying silent or, if anyone asks you what night-times are like, merely stating what the situation is, fairly neutrally. You may have to say quite firmly to some people that you've decided to accept the way things are at the moment and that you may think again when your child is older – but not at present.

It will help you to stick to all this if you can share the job of comforting and caring for your child at night with your partner, and if you both share the same view. Also, try to find ways of getting a break from constant childcare day and night.

It might well be right to do nothing about the situation for a number of reasons:

- Your child may have been ill recently, and perhaps been through an uncomfortable and distressing time.
- Your child may have had to be separated from you and may need the reassurance of seeing you always around.
- A major change – such as a house move, or a new sibling, may have affected him.
- There may be other tensions in the family, such as a marital problem, or something distressing may have happened to people close to you.
- Your child may be about to/may have just started playgroup or nursery school.

DOING SOMETHING ...

Broadly, doing something to try and aim for a better night's sleep for everyone means a choice of three options:

1. Leaving your child to cry, sometimes called 'crying it out'.
2. Sharing your bed with your child, sometimes known as 'the family bed'.

Toddlers and Pre-schoolers

3. The checking method, sometimes called 'teaching in small steps'.

It's difficult to see how you could combine any one or two or three of these options, as success in these situations does depend on consistency and predictability. Stick with what you choose, or you will make very little difference.

Leaving your Child to Cry

I know loving, caring parents who have done this and had no regrets, sometimes with young babies. It has also been advocated as a method for dealing with babies of just a few weeks old who cry a lot[3] by a paediatrician who admits babies and toddlers into a hospital ward to cure their crying (and sleeplessness), if necessary. One of the best-selling and well-established childcare books puts it forward as part of everyday child management.[4] It was one of the main methods of child-rearing outlined in the works of the very influential New Zealand doctor Truby King in the 1930s and 40s. He was strongly pro-breastfeeding at a time when artificial feeding was beginning to make headway, but didn't believe in feeding too often or feeding at night, and felt babies should be taught to 'go without' by being left to cry.

It fits in with our society's comparatively recent idea (in terms of human evolution) that babies and children should be separated as quickly as possible from anyone they might be dependent on. It fits in with notions of discipline, of parents laying down the law and feeling that any challenge to their rules needs to be sat upon.

These points are, to me, the method's downside.

But there is an idea, if not an actual philosophy, behind this approach. It is that giving your baby or child attention in the night actually encourages him to wake up and call for you – and by taking away that 'reward' you encourage him to learn to stay asleep and/or to get himself back to sleep when he wakes.

How to Get a Good Night's Sleep

There is some support for the notion that you can stimulate an infant too much when he is distressed, and exacerbate a problem. Parents can get themselves on a treadmill, giving more and more attention and getting more and more desperate in the attempt to settle and soothe their infants. This is the explanation given for the fact that babies who have been admitted to hospital for crying (when organic causes have been ruled out) do tend to improve.[5] In hospital a crying baby doesn't receive the winding, cuddling, rocking, patting and play, he gets at home if he shows distress. This allows the baby or child to develop his own strategies for calming himself, and this in turn allows sleep (*for more on this, see page 66–67*).

Other parents feel that if a child cries in the night, he needs comfort.

Iona:

My mother has always said we were spoiling our children, going to them when they cried. She calls it 'giving in to them'. Now that both of them wake up and cry out several times a night, she feels she's been proved right. But there's never been a time when I've felt I could just leave them to cry. It just doesn't feel right to do it. If I hear a cry, I don't immediately get anxious – but I am aware it can mean someone's unhappy, and that it's my role to sort things out if I can. If that means taking either of them into bed with us, then so be it.

Pauline:

I can stand listening to her cry for about two minutes and then I have to go in to check she hasn't hurt herself ... more than that I can't bear.

Maureen:

I have tried to let her cry — she's 20 months old and a terrible sleeper. But she cried and cried one night for two hours. Then she fell asleep exhausted. I said to my husband, 'I can never let that happen again.' It's not fair on anyone — least of all her.

But for other parents, leaving a child to cry is acceptable, as long as they feel they've done what needs to be done to make sure the child is comfortable and not at any risk.

Ollie:

I always put David in his cot after a bath, after a last bottle, in a clean nappy and after a nice, quiet cuddly session together with a book and some songs. If he cries, I know there can be nothing really the matter with him, so I feel confident he has no really good reason for crying.

Note:
If you do decide to leave your baby to cry, try and work out a method of being able to take a peek at your baby without him spotting you. I have heard of a case where a baby got his arm through the bars of the cot and caught his clothing on the screw mechanism that pulled the sides up and down. This should not be possible on a new-style cot, but even if you are sure your baby's cot is safe, there can still be physical reasons, possibly dangerous ones, why your baby might cry. It's best to be in a position to check, unobtrusively.

What You Do
- Choose a time such as a long weekend when you are under less pressure than normal.

- Explain to anyone who might be disturbed by the noise just what you are going to do.
- Check out that you and your partner agree that now's the right time, and that you both feel able to carry it through with perfect consistency.
- Make sure you have in place a quiet, routine winding down-time to bedtime, which also gives you the chance to explain to your child, as far as you can, what you intend to do.
- When your child cries, you do nothing (except perhaps the secret check outlined above).
- You continue to do nothing. Eventually your child will fall asleep, exhausted or convinced you are not going to come to him.
- You continue this for as many nights as it takes to work, and as many times in the night as necessary.

Although I do have a personal reluctance about actually advocating or promoting this method, I have known it to work very well, and within just a handful of nights ... if by working well you mean the child stops waking up and crying. A child who feels loved and cared for can learn to be on his own at night, perhaps at some child-like level rationalizing it in some way – that when it's dark and quiet, it is time to be alone, and that nothing awful happens as a result. The old habits die and new ones of sleeping through are set up in their place, with the child simply forgetting what used to happen and what his old expectations were.

The results are fairly quick, and if the trouble starts again you can repeat the method in the same way, to get the same result.

A variation on this method, which some parents may feel is more acceptable and less 'harsh', is to go into the child's room once, *immediately* he starts to cry, and speak firmly and clearly to him, soothing him and reassuring him very briefly without actually taking him out of his cot or bed or allowing him to initiate any contact or conversation. This may well have an advantage of flexibility, especially for children who don't usually wake or cry in the night.

Patsy:

> When I babysit for my nephew, who's three, he always shouts out for me and starts to cry when he's in bed. I think he's just testing me out — and maybe checking I am still there looking after him. He normally has a calm night, according to his mum. I go up, stick my head round the door and say in a very strict voice, 'Now you have to go back to sleep, Peter — I'm just downstairs.' Then I shut the door, and make sure he can hear me going down the stairs.

Sharing the Bed

Worldwide, it is the norm for families to sleep in the same space and for infants and small children to sleep very close to their mothers. This is linked with lengthy (by our standards) breastfeeding, and with feeding babies on demand, day and night, until well beyond the first or even second year of life. The child's place next to his mother may be taken by the next youngest child rather than by social norms that encourage him into his own room and bed.

Many families have their baby in the same room as them while the baby is very small. There's sound sense in this, we now know, as it seems to offer protection against cot death — parents become more aware of their baby's normal and abnormal noises and snuffles at night (though, tragically, babies can die lying next to their parents, and even sleeping or feeding in their parents arms). The Foundation for the Study of Infant Deaths recommends parents to have their babies sleeping in the same room for at least the first six months. According to some experts it could be that the comparatively low cot death rate among Asian populations is connected to their practice of sleeping with their infants (*for more on cot death, see pages 46 and 81*).

Sharing the actual parental bed is something that causes more controversy.

The old worry of 'overlying', sometimes actually used on death certificates of babies in the past, is related to fears that the sleeping or drowsy parent could roll over and suffocate the sleeping baby. These days, deaths in these circumstances would probably be classified as a cot death once other causes had been eliminated.

It does seem that cot death is linked with overheating, and a vulnerable baby's inability to deal with his rise in body temperature. It's this genuine concern that has caused some professionals to advise parents not to take their babies into bed with them — the increased heat caused by the parents' bodies, plus the possibly heavy bedding on the adult bed, could be too much. It also seems sensible to advise against any bed-sharing if you or your partner has been drinking heavily or takes medication in order to sleep. A deep, heavy sleep may mean you won't wake up if your baby cries because he's uncomfortable, and it could, in theory at any rate, mean you could roll over onto your baby without waking yourself up.

Ask your health visitor about it, and give yourself the opportunity to talk this issue through. It would seem a sensible compromise to feed and sleep with your baby in your bed if you want to — and it is a loving, warm, close feeling to have a tiny baby snuggled up against you, and one I look back on with pleasure now my children are older — but to keep your baby on the outside edge of the bed, and to make sure any bedding isn't wrapping your baby up too tight. Perhaps your baby needs no clothing other than a vest and a nappy when he's in bed with you, rather than the sleep suit you might dress him in if he was in his own cot away from you.

Toddlers and Pre-schoolers

Choosing the Family Bed

Some families decide to share a bed from the start, or to make it a positive choice if sleep problems arise with their child.

It helps if you have a larger-than-double-size bed. If you don't want to buy a new bed, two single beds pushed together is a substitute, but a second-best one according to families who have tried both, especially if you have a child who moves around a lot in bed or who's a restless sleeper. Another alternative is a futon or a large mattress on the floor. Some families drop the side of the cot nearest the big bed and adjust the base to a level with the bed – again, it's not as satisfactory a solution as a 'proper' queen- or king-size bed.

Fans of bed-sharing say it brings the family closer together, and that being together at night is cozy, comfortable and loving.

If you want to have sex with your partner, you can go to a different room. Some parents move the sleeping child to another room instead, knowing that if the child is deeply enough asleep he's unlikely to wake while being moved. You'll have to work out your own best arrangements; some children would certainly wake up if they were put somewhere else.

Children who know they are welcome in the big bed, and feels it's as much their space as their parents, tend to graduate to their own room and bed at about three or four. They may then continue to come into the big bed in the middle of the night. The next stage is that they come in when feeling poorly, frightened or lonely, until the majority of most nights are spent in their own room and their own bed. Some families have a roll-up mattress and a sleeping bag on hand in their room, so the child can use this instead of actually climbing in with them.

Pauline:

> Both our children have slept with us from being babies. Our younger child is now 18 months, and is still in with us. Our first child is four and sleeps most nights on her own, as she has done

for about a year. We had to get a bigger bed when the baby was born, as four of us just couldn't sleep comfortably in the double bed which we'd managed with until then.

When our four-year-old was coming up to her third birthday, we started suggesting she try her own bed sometimes — she already had a room with a bed in, where her clothes and some of her books and toys were kept. But it was her choice where she slept, and she knew that. However, we did encourage her when she went into her bed the odd time, I suppose. She built up from that, and only comes in to us if she wakes up having had a bad dream or if she feels a bit unwell — and even then she often trots back to her own room after a cuddle.

A variation on bed-sharing is to start off the night with your child and then take him back when he is deeply asleep. Or you can accept him into your bed after he starts off in his own. Other parents take it in turns to get into bed with the child, though this can be uncomfortable if the child has a single bed. The point of whatever you do is to accept it as a positive choice, and one which responds to what your child needs at the moment. You also need to know it won't last forever — and you always have the option of teaching your child new ways of settling and staying settled if you decide it's gone on too long for you to accept.

The Checking Method

This method involves teaching your child to settle himself when he wakes, without disturbing you.

The idea behind it is that a child wakes up and cries for attention when he needs to get back to sleep but can't without the right sort of triggers. You then need to help him learn that different sorts of triggers, or none at all, can be supplied without you being there — but because you can't expect him to learn this

Toddlers and Pre-schoolers

straight away, or simply by being told, you demonstrate it to him in a very practical way. This is done without letting him feel abandoned or neglected.

Basically, you need to change your reactions every time your baby cries out for you, comes downstairs or into your bed, or does whatever he does to gain your attention at night.

You may be in the habit of giving him a breastfeed, a bottle-feed, a cuddle, a play session or a spell in bed with you.

With this method you do none of that. Instead, you soothe your baby with the absolute minimum of attention each time. If he wakes up and cries, you go in after a few minutes (I'd suggest three or four; you may want to go in after just a minute or so – but don't leave it longer than about 10 or 15, or your child could get very distressed indeed). You speak quietly and firmly, but not angrily, say 'goodnight'...and then you leave. You repeat this as often as you need to for your child to accept that you mean what you say, and that you are not going to go through previous settling rituals. Eventually, your child will fall asleep.

You need to repeat this the next night, and the next, and the next ... it may take a week or so before the method gives you an unbroken night, and you may have to get up to check your child many, many times. Some families find it works a lot more quickly than they would have thought, however, and they only need to go into their child two or three times.

You do need to be consistent – and that goes for anyone looking after your child. If you give in, you are back to square one; you will have to begin the programme all over again, perhaps after a short break, and regard it as a new beginning.

It may be that your settling rituals have become very complicated and lengthy, and you may find it hard to believe you could go from these to a simple 'goodnight.' You may even feel bad about making your child cry and beg for you to lie down, or feed him, or play. You are the best judge of this – no one should suggest anything that makes you feel like a bad or cruel parent. You may want a halfway house whereby you gradually reduce the rituals so they work their way down to the 'goodnight' stage.

Phil:

Alex was two and a half and still needing me to go into his bed, lie down and stroke his forehead before he would go back to sleep – maybe twice a night. This could take up to half an hour each time, and I found it hard to get some sleep while I was settling him. I felt I needed more sleep, but I didn't want to make Alex feel bad. So I stroked his forehead for about five minutes, while sitting in a chair by his bed, holding his hand. Then I went back to my bed. I followed that by just sitting in the chair, then I began to move the chair further away...until I was able to calm him by putting my head round the door very briefly, saying 'go back to sleep, Alex. See you in the morning.' One night I just called this out to him through the door, and then after that he started to sleep through. The whole process took about three weeks.

Whatever you do, it helps to keep a diary in which you record the timing and frequency of your child's waking so you can see more clearly any progress. You'll see if the time spent asleep gets longer, and the periods spent crying get shorter.

It also helps to combine this with a regular bedtime routine (*see page 22–26*) which you can adapt to suit your child's needs. By this age, your child doesn't need to be asleep before he gets into bed or into his cot. Putting him in awake, but rested and calm, is good practice for teaching him to settle without you. You may need to reduce the sort of rituals you have for settling him at bedtime: it's fine to have a short sequence of events leading up to kissing your child goodnight and then leaving him to fall asleep on his own, but don't let your child complicate them. Kissing a teddy or two is OK, but some toddlers develop a need to see you kiss all the soft toys on the shelf and in the cupboard, and in a certain way, too, or you have to start again.

If your child asks you to lie down until he goes to sleep, resist

Toddlers and Pre-schoolers

this, copying Phil's gradual distancing approach (*see previous page*) if you prefer. Sometimes, telling your child you are going to do something specific seems to help – just say you are going downstairs to make a cup of coffee and you'll bring it up again with you in a minute, for example. You must keep your promise, even though chances are your child will be asleep by the time you return. After a few occasions, you can drop the promise to return. It's as if it's comforting enough for your child to be able to picture where you are and what you are doing.

You can try this approach from the age of around six to eight months, though it's most popular with parents of toddlers from the age of a year or so up – before then many parents are less than sure their child has a 'good' reason for waking up, and lack the confidence to put the programme into action.

Key Points to Remember
- Be consistent.
- Get your partner's support and share the 'checking' duties.
- Combine the settling programme with a consistent bedtime routine.
- Keep a record of night-time wakings to observe progress.

ENDNOTES
1. G. Scott and M. P. N. Richards, 'Night waking in one-year-old children in England', *Child care health and development* 1990; 16: 283–302.
2. N. Richman *et al.*, 'Behavioural problems in three-year-old children: an epidemiological study in a London borough', *Journal of Child Psychology and Psychiatry* 1975; 12: 5–33.
3. Dr C. R. Jayachandra, *Screaming babies – certainly curable!* (JC Publications).
4. Dr Christopher Green, *Toddler Taming* (Vermilion, 1988).
5. S. McKenzie, 'Troublesome crying in infants: effect of advice to reduce stimulation', *Archives of Disease in Childhood* 1991; 66: 1416–20.

5

Night-time and Its Terrors . . .

Most of us as adults still know what it's like to have a bad dream, or to wake up still frightened from a nasty dream experience that feels as real as anything that happens in the day. Those first few seconds wondering if what you've just been through really did happen are pretty unpleasant and disorientating.

It's not surprising that children can become just as upset as adults, and even more confused, as they are still only beginning to appreciate the full difference between reality and imagination.

Dreams are most likely to happen during what is termed REM sleep. REM stands for rapid eye movement, which has been noted during the medium-to-light sleeping state that happens four or five times a night, alternating with lighter and deeper periods of sleep.

Frequent, even nightly bad dreams are unusual, but many children go through a stage where they are having nightmares more than just occasionally. Dreams and nightmares are thought to be a way of 'organizing' people, places, events and experiences encountered when awake, and it's not surprising that young children, whose experiences are so often new and unfamiliar, seem to have more dreams, and more vividly disturbing dreams, than adults.

Unless your child's nightmares are unresolved after several weeks, or cause her distress in the day, you can assume she will simply grow out of the problem. Comfort her when she wakes, and talk through the dream in the day if she remembers it –

share her feelings about it and reassure her about what dreams are. Depending on the age of your child, you can talk in terms of imagination and pictures in her head, and how they aren't real in the way other experiences are. There's no good reason for probing her to see what her anxieties are, or for assuming she must have some deep underlying worry, unless she shows other symptoms of distress during the day and if she can't be consoled easily at night. Sometimes you will have a clue about what might be upsetting your child – a big change in her life, a recent death or separation, a frightening film or TV programme, a stay in hospital ... without making too big a deal of it, your 'inside knowledge' of your child can help you say the right things to help her sort out the confusing and worrying aspects of her life. Talking about your child's fears in the day, when she's feeling relaxed and comfortable, may well help to reassure her, and to help her see things are not as frightening as she imagines in the night. Some children are helped by painting or drawing the thing that makes them afraid.

Jill:

Robert was about three when he started having a series of frightening nightmares, usually about things he'd seen on TV – even quite friendly things, like puppets or characters he'd seen in children's programmes reappeared at night in terrifying forms, according to what he said. It turned out when we started talking that he hadn't yet understood about actors and acting in TV programmes, and about the way people dressed up to pretend to be something different. It was a revelation to him when I explained about this – his nightmares stopped soon after.

Sue:

Polly started to wake up crying shortly after she started playgroup. She wasn't able to talk about her dreams — she was only just over two, and not talking very well — but I was sure it was something to do with playgroup that was bothering her, despite the fact she seemed to enjoy going there — the timing was too coincidental. I still can't really explain what was going on in her mind, except they were obviously new experiences and new people she was encountering. I let her come into our bed for a cuddle when she woke up, and I started staying with her at playgroup, just for a few minutes while she got settled in instead of sneaking off before she noticed I'd gone. I honestly don't know if it made any difference, but she settled down shortly after this.

You can encourage your child to have some control over her bad dreams. If she becomes frightened to sleep, or to go to bed because of them, tackle them together. Help her to go to bed thinking of pleasant experiences, bringing to mind some happy memories or some anticipated event. Use your own imagination — if your child wakes up scared of the horrible dragon, imagine it shrinking in size, together, so it finally disappears. Or turn it into a friendly, protective dragon who's keen to look after her. Maurice Sendak's wonderful and classic picture storybook *Where the Wild Things Are* is enthralling for children from about the age of three, and has a reassuring message about bad dreams that could help as well.

Some of the stresses of life we can't do anything about, and we can't always change what goes on in our child's head. We can, however, help her learn to cope with the difficult aspects of life, and teach her that we experience them, too.

Night-time and Its Terrors . . .

FEAR OF GOING TO BED

Toddlerhood and early childhood are times when fears, irrational and rational, are very common among children who are otherwise happy, well-loved and cared for. Fears can be of anything – men with moustaches, dogs, monsters in books and stories, loud noises, fireworks ...

I don't think we can always dismiss toddler fears as being 'normal', although they are certainly a part of their emotional and mental development. Recent and tragic child abuse cases indicate that we do need to listen to what toddlers are trying to say to us, for example, and to take their expressions of distress seriously.

That's my warning note, and please accept that it's not intended to make you assume that any fear your child shows is a symptom of something horrible having happened to her that you don't know about. It is far more likely that your child's fear, while serious enough to her, is an expression of something going on in her head, even if its inspiration has been a real event or an experience that's nothing to do with abuse or violence.

Your child may find that these fears can be coped with in the day when other things are happening and when adults are around to act as a buffer. But at night, alone in the bedroom, the fears can seem overwhelming. A child who has been happy to go to bed for some time may start to resist bedtime and to need company while she falls asleep.

Helen:

Our house was burgled when Kate was aged three. The worst thing was that it was done while we were asleep – and we never knew anything about it until the next morning. This had a very bad effect on Kate, who started to be afraid of going upstairs even during the day. It was worse at bedtime – she didn't really say it was the burglary that had made her afraid, and I'm not even sure if she was able to rationalize it to this extent. I tried to help by showing her that the windows upstairs were properly locked, and that no one could get into the house now we had made the whole place more secure. But I think the fear had got into her quite deeply. It took about three months before the worry gradually subsided. Until then, we just had to deal with it by leaving her bedroom light on, leaving the door open, and letting her hear the noise of downstairs activity ... and by not talking about the burglary in front of her, so as not to remind her.

It can help to make the fear manageable by helping your child to imagine some control over the nasty experience or 'thing' that's bothering her, as suggested above. I've heard of some parents chasing the witch out of the front door every night, or wagging an admonishing finger at the invisible monster that's set to frighten their child as she goes upstairs to bed, telling it in no uncertain terms to behave.

Helen's idea of making links between the bedroom and the family activity downstairs is worth trying. Sometimes, fear at night can be alleviated entirely by making the whole experience less of a lonely one. There is no need whatsoever in my view to discourage the need for a light on, or to forbid leaving the door open. The idea that a child gets to sleep better with fewer distractions and less stimulation is behind this, I suppose, but a worried, anxious child is unlikely to get to sleep easily ... the dark is a potentially frightening place, especially to someone who is liable to think the shape of her dressing gown hanging on the door is the outline of a ghostly apparition.

Socket lights – glow-in-the-dark plugs you put in the electrical socket – give a warm, low light which might be enough to comfort your child. Music from a radio or cassette player – out of reach for safety if it's a younger child – is also comforting.

Night-time and Its Terrors . . .

NIGHT TERRORS

This phenomenon is rather different to nightmares or bad dreams. With a night terror, the sufferer is unable to remember the experience the next day, or even if woken after the episode.

A night terror happens during deep sleep – not REM sleep when we dream, or dream in a way we can remember the following day – and it can be very frightening. Some experts believe it happens when one part of the brain is in the deepest sleeping state while another is aroused and very active, often frighteningly so to the parent. Night terrors have been described as 'disorders of arousal', and they seem to run in families so there may be a genetic component to them.

The child may screech or scream, and even sit up in bed, with a frightened expression on her face and a terrified look in her eyes. A few children actually sleep walk. The reaction on your part should be to wait until the episode has passed and a calm, rested state takes over. You need to watch in case any of your child's movements lead her into any situation where she might hurt herself, of course. Then tuck your child back into bed when it's finished. The whole thing is usually over in less than 10 minutes, though some can go on for up to half an hour or even longer.

Night terrors are reported as being most common in children between the ages of three and eight, and they happen to about five per cent of children, maybe only once or twice, however.

One overview of the literature on night terrors, included in a well-respected book on sleep and children, reports that researchers have found that night terrors can increase in frequency in susceptible children during a period of stress or a difficult period in the family's life.[1] Keeping to a regular sleep schedule may help, as extreme tiredness seems to make terrors worse. Short-term psychotherapy is suggested as a possible help, to enable parents and child to handle stress in new ways.

There is a school of thought that suggests night terrors in rather older children are a sign of unexpressed anger and emotion in the family as a whole – the outlet becoming the night terrors of the child.

Yvonne:

> *When Barnaby was about four, he had about six episodes of what I now realize were night terrors. He did actually walk in his sleep – and it was obviously sleep. His eyes were open all the time. I'd wake up because I'd hear a noise, and would find him in the doorway of our bedroom, just standing there with a staring expression in his eyes. It would give me a terrible fright. He wouldn't move, or talk – just stand there, stock still. Each time, I'd get out of bed, turn him round and sort of half-lead, half-follow him back to bed. By the time he'd reach his bed he'd already be more obviously asleep, and would lay down with his eyes shut. He'd never remember anything about it the next day. He was about to start school at the time, but I never really linked it with that as he seemed to be looking forward to the move.*

ENDNOTES

1. Dilys Daws, *Through the Night* (Free Association Books, 2nd edn, 1993).

6

Getting Help

Many sleep problems can be solved, accepted or dealt with in whatever way you think is right for you by simple measures you decide to adopt and put into practice yourselves – without any outside help or support.

We've already seen that it helps to tackle any issue with consistency and commitment – anyone closely involved in your baby's life needs to be aware of what you intend to do to change (or not change) any sleeping problem, and if they are involved enough to look after your baby at night, they should do what you are doing.

It can be hard, nevertheless (even with the support of those around you) to see what could help, and to stick to a plan or programme ... and to decide whether doing anything now is the right decision.

This is where people outside the family can offer another pair of eyes and ears, and another set of ideas – people who aren't emotionally involved with you or your child, who have experience of working with sleepless or crying children and who have some sympathy with you.

Today there is professional and voluntary help available. It is useful because it comes from people who won't (or shouldn't) sound as if they are judging your skills as a parent, or dismissing your child as 'naughty' or 'just at that age', or belittling your anxieties by saying you are 'overanxious' or 'simply not firm enough'.

How to Get a Good Night's Sleep

Don't be put off if the first time you look for some advice on your child's sleeping habits you get only unhelpful phrase-making like this. If you believe you have a problem you need help with, then press on until you find someone who will take you seriously and give you advice you really can follow.

Rita:

I saw my GP about Helen's sleeping, not because I thought there was anything medically wrong with her but because I didn't know how to get help otherwise. He wasn't very helpful. He more or less implied there was nothing I could do except live with it — but I'd already decided I didn't want to do that, and that's the reason I was sitting in front of him asking him what I should do instead! He said a lot of nine-month-old babies still wake up at night — I said yes, but do they wake up seven or eight times, and need rocking back to sleep again afterwards on each occasion? He actually said, 'Well, if that's what you have to do, you just have to do it...she'll grow out of it some time.' I then asked my health visitor, and she said 'Oh, Dr X isn't very good with sleeping problems...' and then never said anything else to help me either!

Carmel:

My GP was very good. She suggested I speak to my health visitor, and she gave me some good suggestions — such as working out a bedtime routine and sticking to it. She made sure I told my husband what we should do, as well. She didn't try to impose anything on me — we really did work out together what would be the best way to wind Rosie down in the evening. I explained to her I didn't want to stop breastfeeding just yet, and she just accepted this without any criticism. Friends had said I should stop, to give Rosie a chance to get to sleep without it. But the health visitor said I could just cut down on the time I spent feeding, and aim to get to a stage where Rosie wasn't always falling asleep after a feed.

Getting Help

WHAT'S AVAILABLE TO YOU

In the UK, young families are especially well cared for in terms of access to support from health professionals.

You are entitled to the care of a midwife for up to 28 days after the birth of your baby. In practice this means you will be cared for by midwives in hospital and then receive home visits from a community midwife usually up to 10 days after delivery. The community midwife may not visit every day if she feels you have no problems that need this sort of intensive input – or she may visit twice or even more on one day if she decides it would be helpful.

She should give you a number you can call any time you need to speak to a midwife – this might well include times when you feel desperate because you can't get your baby to sleep. This number will get you in touch with whoever is the duty community midwife at that time. Many maternity units are happy to get calls after you've been discharged, and you will be able to speak to a midwife there, too.

Use the number you've been given any time up to 28 days after the birth of your baby. Thereafter, you and your baby are in the care of the health visitor, a nurse (and often a midwife too) who is qualified in health promotion and in supporting the health and general welfare of families with children under five. It's very common for the community midwife to stop visiting at about 10 days, and to hand you over to the health visitor then. The health visitor will probably make a 'primary visit' in the first 14 days or so, and tell you when and where baby clinic sessions are held.

Your health visitor can become a good source of up-to-date information on child health and development, including sleep problems. She can't actually give your child any medical treatment, but she can tell you when it might be helpful to see the clinic doctor or your GP.

Some health visitors have developed a special interest in

children's sleep. This is mainly because they have become so very aware of how common sleep-related problems are among the parents they visit, and because it is exactly the sort of area, involving counselling and family support, that health visitors are experienced in.

Your family doctor (GP) is another source of information and help – though it has to be said that medics in general, and family doctors in particular, are not usually especially well trained in handling children's sleep problems. Your GP's advice may depend more on his or her own experience and whether he or she has a special interest in the subject. However, your doctor can rule out any underlying organic cause of sleep disturbance or excessive night-time crying, thereby leaving the field clear for other remedies. If you are at all worried that there may be some clinical reason for your child's behaviour, you will of course want to get this checked out first.

Your GP can be the gateway to other services available in your area, and can refer you to other professionals. Your health visitor may be able to do this, too. It's always worth asking your health visitor or doctor if there is anyone in the area offering a 'sleep clinic' service, which may need a professional's referral.

Sleep Clinics

These are not very common, but they are probably more numerous than they were a few years ago.

A typical sleep clinic will be run once a week or more in the outpatient's department of a hospital or in a community health clinic. It may have a number of health professionals involved in it, or just one. There may be some research being done with the people and families who use the services. If your situation is being used for research purposes, then of course you should be informed, and assured of all confidentiality in any published results.

Newcastle upon Tyne has a sleep clinic headed by Glenda

Getting Help

Brown, a health visitor with many years of experience and a special interest in helping families with sleepless children. Parents who come to her are usually referred by their own health visitors and doctors.

'I see parents driven to the brink of desperation by a wakeful toddler,' says Mrs Brown. 'Often, they have lost confidence in their own ability to deal with the situation, and that's why the intensive support offered after the visit to the clinic is so vital.'

Mrs Brown sees parents, one or both, or sometimes a grandparent as well (especially if the grandparent sometimes puts the child to bed) for an initial consultation, which can take half an hour to an hour.

During this time she gets a thorough history of the situation, in order to get the fullest possible picture of the length of time the problem has been going on, and what effects it has had. This time is important for the parents, too, not just as a means of getting the details across, but also as a way of sharing the load with someone who is prepared just to listen, ask relevant questions, and show support – not leaping in with a pat solution, platitudes, or judgments.

Mrs Brown assures the majority of parents that the sleep problem is curable – but that it may not be easy in the first nights to put the cure into practice. She writes down an agreed plan, after discussion with the parents. This plan is likely to involve a daytime and a bedtime routine which fits in with what the family feel able to do, as well as some form of 'checking' method (*see page 48*) which greatly reduces the amount of stimulation and attention the child has been having up until now when he wakes. The length and timing of naps may be adjusted to make more of a settled, predictable sleep routine during the day, too.

One suggestion which can make for a big change is the adjustment to a quieter winding-down part of the pre-bedtime routine. Sometimes, parents with a wakeful child try to exhaust the child in the afternoon and evening, with a round of activities and outings. This is an attempt to tire the child out so he will settle easily and fall into a deep sleep. It rarely works – in fact, it can have the opposite effect, serving to excite the child to a point where he finds it harder, not easier, to settle. It also means that going to bed means he's missing out on all the action ... and for some children, that's a cause of resentment.

The parents are asked to re-read the whole programme carefully and to talk over when they would like to start the programme. There may be some alterations they want to make to the suggestions, too. Mrs Brown normally gets in touch with the family's health visitor, to explain about the sleep programme and to arrange for her to keep in daily contact with the family once the programme is underway.

'That sort of ongoing support is essential,' she explains, 'as it helps families to stick to the plan, knowing they have someone they can talk over successes and difficulties with the next day.'

Mrs Brown also stays in touch, and there is likely to be a repeat visit at the clinic at some stage.

Much of the support is centred on encouraging the parents to regain their confidence in knowing what to do – tiredness, and the way the sleeplessness and settling difficulties seem to get worse rather than better over time, can reduce their self-esteem to the point where they find it difficult to trust their own judgement. Having someone outside the family to share the problem and bolster their determination to do something about it allows them to rebuild this vital confidence and to enjoy a new, rewarding relationship with their child.

'I always say that the parents who bring their children here are loving, caring parents,' says Mrs Brown. 'None of the children are in any way neglected or deprived of love or attention. But [the parents] feel so guilty because they have reached a stage where they resent their son or daughter, and they hate the fact that they can't like them all the time.'

Mrs Brown believes that a sleep and settling programme helps parents see they can set limits and can distance themselves physically from their children without that meaning they are in any way distancing themselves emotionally. The result is an enhanced, even closer relationship than before with their children, with each party knowing what's expected of them, and no one being manoeuvred into a situation they don't want.

Sometimes a child who is finally getting the amount of uninterrupted sleep he needs becomes a happier person to have around, less tetchy and much more pleasant company. Depending on the age of the child, Mrs Brown encourages a nap (or at least a quiet time) at some stage in the day. Sometimes parents with a wakeful child deliberately try not to arrange a daytime sleep in the belief that the child will 'save up' his sleep needs for the night. It rarely works like that, she says. Instead, a daytime sleep can reinforce the settling and sleeping pattern of the night, with the parent or carer placing the child in his cot or bed while he is still awake, and repeating the firm and simple words 'go to sleep now' or 'goodnight, see you soon' they've begun using as part of the night-time routine.

Often, by the time they reach Mrs Brown or any other sleep clinic or counsellor, parents say they have tried everything to get their child to sleep through the night. They will have received a whole load of advice, not all of it requested, and been made to feel sometimes guilty and inadequate, sometimes cruel, sometimes highly anxious about whether the problem indicates something seriously wrong with their child, something that may go on for years to come. The sleep problem may have been the focus of many arguments between mother and father, between the grandparents of the child and the parents, etc. They are by now keen to work with a programme that helps them get back into the driving seat while allowing them to adapt to, and respond to, the needs of their child.

Hospital Stays

Taking a baby or toddler into hospital to 'teach' him a better sleeping pattern does seem a drastic measure. It can't be cheap and, on the face of it, appears to be a case of a sledgehammer to crack a nut.

However, a child with a sleeping problem is a bigger deal to the family than this analogy implies. The solution may seem sledgehammer-like, but the problem is a huge immovable rock, rather than a nut.

I am aware of hospital 'treatment' being used in sleep problems where there is also the confounding situation of a baby who cries a great deal. I have spoken to parents for whom the treatment has worked better than they could have hoped (*for an example, see page 74*).

One factor that I would guess is a crucial one is that bringing the baby into hospital is in itself a powerful acknowledgement that there is indeed something worth complaining about. So many parents say 'no one understands' or 'people think we're making a fuss about nothing.' Sympathy and someone taking you seriously enough to intervene on your behalf – someone who is in addition able to give you a real break from the problem – has a lot going for it.

One approach (*see note on page 51*) purports to cure screaming, sleepless babies by bringing them into hospital and reducing parental contact over the next few days to the absolute minimum.

A similar approach was tried with babies who were compared with a control group cared for at home.[1] The babies ranged in age from three weeks to 10 months. Hypothesizing that it was the reduction in stimulation in hospital – where the babies are routinely ignored if they cry unless there is thought to be something 'wrong' – that causes the lessening of crying, the researchers reckoned that something parents do to a crying baby makes the situation worse. They wondered if the patting, rubbing, winding, rocking and so did not actually reinforce the crying. (Note: while the subjects of this study were undoubtedly crying rather than sleepless babies, I am assuming that these babies hardly slept, either. Observation tells us that the two phenomena go hand in hand.)

The babies studied were either admitted to hospital or their parents were given sympathetic support – by means of an 'empathetic interview' – and advice to reduce stimulation when their baby cried. Babies in both groups improved to the same extent.

The conclusion we can draw from this study is that parents do need support, and that it can be given in the community, i.e. away from hospital, with equally effective results on the behaviour of their children. It could be that this is the crucial factor, rather than the reduction of stimulation – after all, there was no attempt to measure whether or not the advice given to the 'at-home' parents on lessening stimulation had actually been followed.

Thus, acknowledgment and sympathy can be had by means other than having to separate parents and children; family members and friends who offer babysitting services or other ways of giving the parents an occasional break can help to resolve a sleeping problem just as well as a stay in hospital.

Medical Treatment

My impression is that the use of drugs to get babies to sleep used to be a lot more common than it is now. I was more aware of doctors intervening with a prescription 15 or even 10 years ago than I am now.

Of course, tranquillizing babies and children goes back a long way – the most potent 'remedies' were sold over the counter in the last century and in the early years of this one, containing laudanum (a form of opium), alcohol and goodness knows what else. I have heard of mothers these days being advised by their doctor as well as their own mothers and grandmothers to put a drop of whisky in the bottle, or even to give it to the baby on a spoon. None of these remedies is safe.

Drugs used to help a baby get to sleep are not normally the same as 'sleeping pills' prescribed for adults. Usually they are antihistamines, a side-effect of which is drowsiness.

Your doctor will probably not be keen on prescribing anything long term. He or she is likely to give a short course of a drug, to give you a break (if the drug works, and it may well not). No drug is a substitute for deciding on some other way of tackling the situation.

A few parents have found intervention in the form of cranial osteopathy helpful. This involves the manipulation – by someone qualified to do so, I stress – of the bones of the skull. The principle behind it is that being born has given the baby a headache because of the way the skull bones have been misaligned. The result is distress and poor sleep. The remedy involves gently putting the skull back to rights. This method has had its successes (*see page 74*).

Psychotherapy

It is not always easy to obtain psychotherapeutic help for families everywhere, but it is always worth asking your doctor or contacting your local child or family guidance centre for information.

Psychotherapy is sometimes described as 'talking therapy' and it's true that it involves discussion between the therapist and the client. It's more than counselling, however, as the therapist has a profound understanding, or a desire to understand, how past experiences might sometimes mould a person's current outlook, expectations and relationships. He or she is also skilled at helping clients reach insights about themselves.

Psychotherapy can be contrasted with behavioural therapy, which focuses on what the client is actually doing and which attempts to change behaviour more than actually understand it. In terms of this book, sleep clinics as I've described them offer a behavioural approach as they are likely to make suggestions based on an attempt to change what the parent and the child are doing.

A psychotherapeutic approach to sleep problems is more concerned with asking what the crying/sleeplessness actually means, what it could be the result of, what the child may be communicating to (or somehow reflecting back at) the parent.

One leading worker in this field is consultant child psychotherapist Dilys Daws, whose book *Through the Night* is a highly practical, warm and understandable account of her approach.[2]

Mrs Daws works with families over a series of perhaps six meetings. She starts with the 'story' of the baby – his background, events before and during pregnancy and the birth, family reactions. She listens to what the parents are saying, and observes how all three interact. Sometimes, she discovers that the baby's waking may reflect some unmet need in the mother. Or that somehow the parents have not learned to 'tune in to' their baby because of some unresolved issue – such as grief, or childhood resentments that have lasted into adult life. She has discovered that a past bereavement, miscarriage, stillbirth and cot death, or even a difficult birth, can have an effect on this early beginning.

Often what Dilys Daws is trying to do involves helping babies and parents separate from each other at the right time, in the right way. She recognizes the needs of all babies for closeness and intimacy and also 'the need at appropriate moments to take steps away from their parents ... in order to begin to grow up'. Events, feelings and previous family relationships can get in the way of this – but once there is some insight, parents can gain confidence in their own ability to understand their children's needs and not to be overwhelmed, bemused or distressed by them.

ENDNOTES
1. S. McKenzie, 'Troublesome crying in infants: effect of advice to reduce stimulation', *Archives of Disease in Childhood* 1991; 66: 1416–29.
2. Dilys Daws, *Through the Night* (Free Association Books, 2nd edn, 1993).

7

'It Worked for Me...'

These stories reflect the wide range of sleep-related problems experienced by families with babies and young children ... and the wide range of their solutions and approaches.

> ### 10-month-old Difficult to Settle
>
> *Tim was 10 months old and still difficult to settle. He had been breastfed until the previous month, when he just lost interest. This meant that there was no longer an easy way to get him to fall asleep in the evening – once he did, though, he would sleep through most nights. But putting him into his cot meant a lot of yelling and tears, and he was in and out of his cot several times before he finally fell asleep, exhausted. He was OK about going in during the day – I think because he was too tired to object. I wasn't keen on waiting an hour or two for him to feel equally tired at night – so we tried the checking method. We put him down in his cot after a quiet time, and simply said 'goodnight' with a last cuddle, and left him. We left the door open a bit so he could hear us and see the light on outside the room. He yelled and cried – he was very cross, as usual.*
>
> *We returned every minute – I couldn't leave him crying longer than that – and said the same thing, without actually picking him up out of his cot. I can still remember his look of surprise when I said 'goodnight' and walked away from him, without*

taking him out. That wasn't what he had in mind at all!

It meant a lot of return visits, but after about a dozen he lay down quietly and within a short time he was asleep. The next night wasn't so bad, and by the third night we only had to go to him a couple of times. We repeated the process a few months later when his settling had become disrupted after we'd been on holiday. I did feel a bit bad, I suppose, leaving him when he so obviously wanted to be out of his cot — but I really enjoyed having free time in the evenings, and I honestly don't think he resented us, or felt unhappy about being left.

Margie

Three-year-old Who Cries and Wakes

Our story is a dramatic one, and it had a dramatic effect on our family when it finally resolved itself. Anthony had always seemed to be an unhappy baby. Nothing I could do would keep him happy for long. He needed constant cuddling, feeding, soothing, for the first six or seven months, otherwise he would cry — sometimes loudly, sometimes more of a whimper. Of course I took him to the doctor, and we were told there was nothing wrong, and that he had colic which he would eventually grow out of. He was gaining weight and developing well, and there was no other sign that all wasn't well.

As time went on, he still seemed miserable for such a lot of the time. I felt incompetent. Why did no one else's child behave like this? I used to feel guilty saying how bad things were, as if I was criticizing Anthony the whole time. It got to the stage where I was embarrassed going out with such a whingeing, whiny child.

Our sex life was a joke — and a distant memory. When I think about it, we felt so disappointed in each other as parents, and disappointed in Anthony. We had been looking forward to being a family so much, and every day was a struggle.

Eventually, someone suggested I take him to a cranial osteopath.

After just one visit, the change in Anthony was remarkable. He was definitely happier. After two more visits, he was a different child. The whole course lasted six sessions, and it utterly transformed us. He cried occasionally, of course, but I could always tell why, and put things right. He stopped waking up as often in the night, and had a regular sleep in the day. I was told that his skull had been put out of alignment during the birth, and when the osteopath manipulated the skull bones, this helped correct it.

Our whole family is so much happier now, and Anthony continues to be a contented, delightful toddler.

Jane

Baby Sleep-trained

We had a difficult first year with our first child, Anna, as she was very wakeful and never really got into a sleep routine until she was about two. When I was pregnant for the second time, we decided to do things differently from the start. Charlie was put in his own room from the start and encouraged to go to sleep at what we felt was a reasonable time from the age of about two months. I had been feeding him at about 10 p.m., and again at about 2 a.m., but we felt he could be encouraged to sleep through by that time. We did this by putting him in his cot awake, and then leaving him. If he cried, we went in after a few minutes to give a quick look to check he was OK, and then we just left. He cried for about half an hour the first night, and about 20 minutes the second and third nights, and after that he just slept without waking until about 6 o'clock the next morning. He's now a year old, and still a good sleeper.

Kate

Note
See *page 45* for more discussion on where the very young baby should sleep.

Crying Baby Helped by Hospitalization

Tania was five months old, and I was sick of people telling me she had colic, or saying she was deliberately winding me up. She just cried and cried the whole time. I knew there wasn't anything seriously wrong with her — she fed well, she was gaining weight, and she looked very healthy. We'd gone from a diagnosis of colic, to one of teething, and then I was told 'she'll grow out of it.'

She wouldn't stop crying for long enough for me to start enjoying her. She only ever took catnaps — never a proper, satisfying sleep. I was at the end of my tether. There were constant family rows about it, and she almost broke up my marriage. We were living with my parents at the time, and the strain on all of us was impossible to cope with.

Then the GP, sick of me begging for something that would stop the crying, I think, referred me and Tania, with my husband, to the paediatrician. For the first time, I felt something could be done about it.

He decided Tania needed to come into hospital...and we must have looked desperate, as he had her admitted the same day we saw him. My feeling was one of relief — someone else was going to share this terrible problem.

I was told I could only visit her for one hour a day. The next day I came in for that visit. I went in, and saw Tania playing in her cot, happy as anything. I'd never seen her looking so contented. Then she looked up and saw me — and cried. I felt terrible.

She had slept through all night in hospital, and continued to do so for the three days she was there. We took her home, and treated her differently. The doctor said we had not 'managed' her well. We had picked her up all the time, and hadn't let her have her own space. I think this was down to the fact there were four adults in the house always ready to cuddle her and rock her and play with her, all desperate to keep her happy. But she wanted more calm, less stimulation. She had been crying with frustration, and hadn't been able to tell me, of course, what she wanted.

The improvement continued when we went home and we never looked back.

Tammy

The Sleep Clinic Helped

Eleanor spent her first nine months in my bed with me. My husband was in the army, and he was away most of that time. When he left the army we tried to change Eleanor's pattern. But she would only go to sleep in the living room, and then not until 11 o'clock. She'd then wake up several times in the night, whether she was in with us or on her own, and she'd demand some sort of attention. We were both getting more and more exhausted.

When she was three, we'd reached the end of the road with her. I broke down in tears in front of the health visitor, and she sent me to a sleep clinic run by one of her colleagues.

It worked really well – we were given a lot of support in deciding how to wind Eleanor down for the evening, and establishing a routine. This made settling her down in her bed a whole lot easier, and a good deal quicker, too. She was old enough to appreciate a bit of bribery, so I bought some stickers and a book for them, and awarded her a sticker for every night she stayed in her bed. If she came into our room, I just calmly took her back – and she didn't get a sticker. She really cottoned on to this idea and she enjoyed her sticker book such a lot. Now I would say she is a good sleeper, and it only took about three weeks from start to finish.

We are so much happier as a family – we used to get so irritable, and shout at each other the whole day. It's so different now.

Julie

The Family Bed

My own feeling is that it's just not worth fighting a wakeful child. We did with our first. The only way for us to have a night's sleep was to accept her in with us, and then we'd put her back in her bed ... and then an hour later she'd be in with us again, and then one of us would get into her bed with her, to allow the other one to have some room to sleep well ... and then we'd try to sneak back into the big bed, without waking the other partner ... and so on. Second time round, we decided that babies probably need to stay close and snuggled during the night, and we wouldn't argue if this coming baby felt the same.

When Christian was born he had a crib, but at night he would sleep with us, right from being a tiny baby. We had a bigger bed by now, and just had him in all night. He seemed to be a much less jumpy sleeper than his sister; he wouldn't toss and turn as she used to, but maybe that's just a coincidence. He is a more placid personality anyway – though there are people who would say he is like this because his nights have always been geared to his needs.

He's now 18 months, and I think I can see a time when he will want his own cot. I won't mind, though I actually like having him in with us.

Patricia

Accepting the Broken Nights

When I look back, maybe there was something I could have done to change the pattern of broken nights. I never felt strongly enough about it, and neither did Paul. I suppose we just kept going on and on, without it getting to the stage where either of us felt we couldn't go on much longer. I know when Jade was a baby she had what I am convinced was colic, and while it was awful, everyone reassured us it would go in time, and it did. By about 10 weeks she was already less difficult to settle, and I thought only getting up twice in the night for a short breastfeed was bliss compared to the hours I had spent without sleep and at my wit's end with worry in case she was in desperate pain.

Then we had a bad patch at about seven or eight months, when she wasn't very well — just coughs and sniffles one after the other for about four weeks. When she got over that and started to settle easily, I thought that was good as well.

She was still waking up regularly at about a year to 15 months, and it was irritating I suppose, as she'd wake just when I'd drifted into a sleep. But again she settled OK if I did the right thing — a breastfeed or a cuddle in bed with us, or sometimes just finding her dummy for her would do.

I sometimes felt people were critical of her continued waking, but I knew loads of other people who had kids waking up a lot more than Jade, and who seemed far more frantic about it than we were. I never really thought about how long it would last ... I suppose both Paul and I assumed she would grow out of whatever it was as she got a bit older. I've never got cross with her about waking, but I've never made a big fuss about it either — at least not since those early weeks when I thought she must be ill.

She did start to sleep through more and more, and the night-time wakings grew less and less frequent. She's now four, and she does sometimes come in with us for a very brief cuddle if she feels lonely or cold or something. But she does it less and less.

Linda

Afraid of the Dark

Natalie was always very good at sleeping through the night, even when she was a tiny baby. So we were puzzled when she started waking up and crying at about 15 months. She would settle down again after about 10 minutes, falling asleep in our arms, but something was obviously bothering her enough to cry out for us.

She couldn't tell us what it was — but I was convinced it was something concrete, and not something like a 'bad habit' she had

> *got into. It wasn't that she was thirsty — she knocked the cup out of our hands if we offered it to her. In the end, I discovered by chance that she just didn't like the dark. We'd always been careful to shut the bedroom door behind us when we left her in her cot so the landing light wouldn't wake her up and to keep her from hearing any noises from downstairs. One night I forgot to shut it properly, and she didn't call out. The next night I deliberately left the door open, and she still didn't disturb us. I can only assume she was frightened if she woke up at night in pitch-black darkness — and that when she woke up and it was lighter, and she was able to reassure herself where she was, she was able to get back to sleep by herself.*
>
> Ros

8

Questions

Here are some of the questions parents often ask ...

Dummies

Do you think dummies are a good idea to help a baby get to sleep?

Many of the objections people have about dummies are snobbish ones – they're supposed to be associated with 'lower' social classes, though for the life of me I can't see why. I've known parents from all different backgrounds who have used them, and been glad to have them!

Babies like to suck, and get a lot of comfort from sucking. It's a powerful instinct, and those who don't have dummies will suck bits of blanket, thumbs, fingers or something else. Many children don't seem to have a long-lasting need of this sort, of course, and just because you don't give your child a dummy doesn't mean he will suck his thumb instead.

Some babies do come to depend on their dummy to get to sleep, and to stay asleep. It's a nuisance to have to get out of bed at night to 'plug in' a lost dummy – whereas a child who sucks a thumb always has it to hand, as it were. However, older toddlers can search and find their dummies themselves, or you can plant a spare one by the cot or bed if necessary. When it comes to getting rid of the dummy – and many families find that, left to himself, their child would cling on for years and years – it's a lot easier to chuck it out or 'lose' it permanently than to discourage finger- or thumb-sucking. Long-lasting digit-sucking can distort teeth. In the end, it's up to you. There are no overwhelming arguments against using a dummy as far as I can see, as long as you introduce it after you have established breastfeeding – if you do it too soon it can 'confuse' the baby's sucking reflex.

PND and Sleep

Can a mother's post-natal depression affect a baby's sleeping pattern? Or can it make a baby cry?

It's difficult to be sure about this, but consultant child psychotherapist Dilys Daws has looked at the literature, and her own observations, and concluded that there is indeed some relationship between a mother's depression after childbirth and her baby's sleeping and crying (*see reference to her book on page 58*).

It could be that the mother's PND affects her ability to tune in to her baby and work out what might soothe him best; it could be that the baby's crying reflects the mother's own distress back to her, and makes her even less able to cope with it.

This is not the same as 'blaming' the mother for her baby's inability to go to sleep or stay asleep ... but it is a way of noting that mother and baby can be part of the same situation, and that the situation may need some unravelling before both 'bits' of it can be helped.

Sometimes, PND can be masked by the fact that the baby cries and doesn't sleep. The focus is on this rather than on the mother's depression – reinforced by the way some mothers with PND don't admit to those closest to them just how dreadful they feel. But if you feel constantly tired, inadequate, as if you're a poor mother compared to others, if you're often tearful and feel everyone else is better at mothering than you, then think about whether PND could be affecting you. And seek help.

Sleeping Position

What's the best way to lay a baby down to sleep? I know the advice has changed in the past few years.

True. When I had my first baby, new mothers were told to lay their babies on their fronts because there was a fear that if a baby vomited while on her back there could be a risk of choking. In the early 1990s, however, research from elsewhere in the world, notably New Zealand, indicated that babies who slept on their backs were less likely to die of cot death, or sudden infant death syndrome. The other factors identified as making a difference were whether or not the parents smoked, whether the baby was bottle-fed, and whether the baby was too hot – all of which appeared to increase the risk of cot death, independent of other social or economic aspects of the baby's background.

In the UK, these points were translated into the 'back to sleep' campaign, although mothers are not told in this campaign about the protective effect of breastfeeding, as the UK Department of Health feels the evidence is not strong enough. Now we're advised that babies should be placed in their cots on their backs – and figures so far indicate that this advice has significantly reduced the cot death rates.

Why this should make a difference is not yet fully understood. It could be that babies are able to cool themselves down more easily and prevent overheating if they are not face down. Some research suggests close contact with the mattress allows the baby to breathe in poisonous fumes produced by chemicals involved in the mattress manufacture. Being face-down may interfere with breathing in vulnerable babies. As time goes on, we are likely to understand the cause of cot death more fully, and many experts feel it will be multi-factorial – caused by many things. In the meantime, it seems essential to follow current advice and to put your baby to sleep on her back or side – and to keep alert for new research which might throw further light on the safety or otherwise of cot mattresses.

Breastfeeding – for Longer than 'Normal'

I've been told that I am adding to my child's sleep problem by continuing to breastfeed him. He's 17 months, and although I never really envisaged feeding him for this long, it's just happened this way. It's the one thing that gets him back to sleep efficiently and quickly. He wakes two or three times in the night, cries out and I go to him straight away, to stop him getting too loud and waking up my husband. I give him a feed lasting about 10 minutes, during which time he falls back into a sound sleep. I

can then put him back into his cot and get back into bed myself. I have tried to get him to go to sleep without a feed, and my husband has tried to settle him – but he just goes frantic and takes longer to settle in the end, even with a breastfeed. Should I just stop, and refuse to feed him in the night, weathering the storm until he gets the message? Or is he likely to carry on wanting to have breastmilk until he's a lot older? At the moment he feeds during the night and last thing in the evening – and only very occasionally during the day.

This is such a personal situation, depending on you and your feelings, that it's hard to advise you. I think your son is in the situation of not being able to get himself back to sleep when he wakes in the night. Instead of only half-waking and then settling himself back to sleep without disturbing you – which is what most 'good sleepers' actually do – he wakes up 'properly' and is unable to sleep again without a breastfeed. Giving him the breastfeed doesn't help him develop the strategies to get back to sleep himself – but I can quite understand that it is a quick way to settle him, and one which has the virtue of being minimally disturbing to you and your husband. It depends how badly you want to have an uninterrupted sleep – probably you feel you can put up with the waking and getting out of bed most of the time, but it may be a nuisance some of the time, especially when you're already tired, or if it's a cold night.

You need to know that toddlers sometimes do get keener on the breast as they progress through their second year. I know of no good figures on this, but observation strongly suggests that this is the case. It's not uncommon to find that a toddler who has long had no feeds in the day starts asking for them, and becomes less easy to distract from this as he gets better at insisting on what he wants. This doesn't matter a jot, of course, unless you would prefer not to have this happen. Stopping the breastfeeds at night is one step you can take to pre-empt this – and it is likely, if you can be consistent and stick to it, that your child's nights will improve.

Pick a time when you feel strong enough to stick to your guns. Involve your husband, and explain why you feel it's a good time to nip breastfeeding in the bud. When your son wakes, go to him and settle him without getting him out of his cot, and then leave him – following the checking method (*page 48*). You may need to remind yourself that your son doesn't need the breastmilk from a nutritional point of view (I'm presuming he has a good and varied diet through the day). If you think he could be thirsty, he can have a cup of water (have one ready in the room to offer him).

Keep the evening feed going for the moment. It's not a good idea to stop feeding suddenly when you are used to giving three to four feeds in 24 hours, though it's likely you are making very little in terms of volume. You may get uncomfortably full, none the less, if you stop too quickly.

If you don't feel you want to stick to breaking his night-time feeding habit – and it could take a few nights before it 'works' – then don't feel you've 'failed'. Try again another time, if you want to, or just leave it up to your child to stop when he's ready...whenever this might be. Weaning older toddlers from the breast may call for other strategies, involving language and persuasion, which you can't really use with a younger child.

Early Waking

My daughter is two, and she still wears a nappy at night. The problem I have with her is early waking – she wakes up at about 5.30 every morning with a dirty nappy. She doesn't use the toilet for her bowel motions and, I think, relies on the fact she has a nappy on at night to avoid it. I always get up to change her nappy, as she has a tendency to nappy rash which I think would get worse if she was left in the nappy. Of course then she's ready for getting up, as lively as anything ... and she won't go back into her cot for anything. Have you any ideas on how to change her pattern?

From what you say, your daughter is used to going without a nappy in the day. It could be that you might help her do without one at night, now. Sometimes, between the ages of two and three, children respond well to going without the night nappy, and either 'hang on' all night without waking up, or else their full bladder wakes them sufficiently to get up and use the loo. Think about whether your daughter would be ready for this.

If you try this for a few nights you may find she responds well, but she may need your help to use the toilet if she still wakes up wanting to open her bowels. Chances are her habits will change, though, and you can encourage her (with lots of praise, even a small reward) to use the toilet. Make sure she is quite comfortable on the toilet – a small box or stool to rest her feet on will avoid the feeling of being 'perched' which so many children dislike, and which makes them feel they might even fall in. She may prefer to use a potty for her bowel motions for a while, and this is fine if it can build her confidence. Some parents have found they can help overcome their child's reluctance to use the potty and not a nappy for a bowel motion by placing a nappy in the bottom of the potty, opened out, so the child is sitting on the nappy, not the potty – it may sound daft, but it seems to work, as the child still feels she is almost wearing the nappy.

Take heart, though, from the fact that your daughter is almost certain to grow out of this reluctance to use the potty or toilet, and if this is the only thing that's making her wake up, the early waking will probably go as well. In the mean time, if you decide to carry on with the situation as it is, make early mornings low key and boring; keep conversation to a minimum and don't switch on a bright light or draw the curtains if it's dark. Explain to your daughter that it's still night-time – and calmly and firmly put her back to bed with a clean nappy on. If you stick to this, she'll get the message and may make up her mind to go back to sleep, or at least lie down quietly.

Wind at 15 Months

No one believes me when I say this, but I am absolutely sure that my daughter still suffers from wind even though she is now 15 months old.

I am convinced it's this that's waking her up at night. I sometimes see her before she wakes, and she is wriggling round, moaning and screwing her face up – and I know before long she'll be

awake, crying and then screaming if I don't go to her straight away. I can hear the air in her tummy making noises when I cuddle her. Sometimes she gets rid of the wind as I pick her up, and she calms down as I hold her and talk to her. When she's settled I put her back in her cot and she's happy to be left – until she wakes up again. This happens at least once a night.

She had colic very badly when she was a baby, and my doctor advised colic drops, which seemed to help a bit. Now, however, they don't seem to do her any good and my doctor says categorically, 'Babies of this age don't get wind.'

Should I see if there's something in her diet that's giving her a problem?

I think you'll find most doctors are sceptical of wind in toddlers – but there's no logical reason for accepting it exists in young babies yet refuting its existence in older ones.

I have to say, though, that I think it's more likely that your daughter is waking up and needing you to settle her because of a habit rather than as a result of any physical cause. It's normal for babies to wriggle and moan a bit in their sleep from time to time, and you may just be observing your daughter as she goes through that REM stage of sleep which is lighter and more susceptible to disturbance than deeper stages. Your daughter wakes up and then cries and even screams because she needs to get back to sleep again, but can't on her own.

Crying in itself causes babies to take in air – and the noises you hear can be heard in everyone's tummy if you listen! It's also normal for her to release some wind as you move her.

Before making any changes to her diet – and if you decide to do this, do check with your health visitor first – try the 'checking' method of settling (see page 48). Get your doctor's support, if you like, so you can feel convinced that you're not harming your daughter or leaving her in pain.

No More Bottles

My son is 14 months old and he still has a couple of bottles of milk when he wakes in the night. He seems to need them as he drains every last drop, then goes back to sleep quite contentedly.

I now learn that it's not a good idea to give milk or to give bottles to babies of his age, but I have no idea how to stop him needing the bottles. He only has bottles in the day with meals and he will happily use a cup from time to time.

How can I wean him from these bottles?

You're right about the disadvantages of bottles – but the ones your son has in the day don't pose a problem because he is having them with his meals. It's the 'all-day-swigging-bottle' that can affect teeth, because it means the mouth is bathed in liquid for much of the day (water would be OK, but how many toddlers accept a bottle of water?) The bottles your son has when he wakes at night aren't all that risky to his teeth, as he is draining them and then leaving them – he isn't falling asleep with a teat full of milk remaining in his mouth.

Nevertheless, he shouldn't really need this amount of milk – and it could be interfering with his intake of other foods in the day. He doesn't need more than a pint of milk (at the absolute most) at his age, and if he's having too much it could reduce his appetite for a wide range of other foods with other nutrients. It's also likely that he has come to associate the milk with a 'reward' for waking up and crying out.

One way of reducing his need for the bottles, if you don't want to stop suddenly, is to make the milk less attractive. Gradually dilute it more and more with water – go carefully, so he doesn't notice – and reduce its volume by small amounts over a period of several nights. The idea is that he will regard it as less and less of a prize. In the end, though, I would guess you will have to bite the bullet and simply refuse to give him a bottle at night. Soothe and calm him and offer him a cup of water, if you want to, and check him every few minutes until he learns to get himself back to sleep without needing this help. Be prepared for his appetite to increase in the day.

Falling Asleep at the Breast

My baby is six weeks old, and I am breastfeeding him. I have been told it's not a good idea to let him fall asleep at the breast, so he learns how to do it himself without becoming 'hooked' on the need to suck to sleep. However, I find it really hard to do this.

Questions

Sometimes he just falls asleep without me spotting he's about to do it. His eyes are often closed when he's feeding, anyway, then he just comes off, looking very full, and obviously quite deeply asleep. I have tried to get in there in the moments before I think he's about to 'go' ... but he just cries and I have to put him back on the breast again. Am I right to worry about what I'm doing?
I don't think so. It's normal for babies to fall asleep when they have had enough to eat and, as you say, sometimes they reach that stage without any warning. The baby pushes the teat out of his mouth, or comes off the breast, very naturally and spontaneously. Trying to anticipate this is difficult and, as you've found, it can lead to the baby being upset and frustrated.

Older babies can reach a stage when they are able to fall asleep *only* by sucking – it is then that parents are sometimes advised to help them learn other ways of getting to sleep. But a younger baby doing this is only doing what comes naturally, and it doesn't mean you are 'allowing' him to indulge in 'bad habits'. Your baby needs to feed according to his appetite, in order to grow and develop and to help you to establish a reliable, plentiful milk supply. At his age it's just that appetite, feeding, contentment and sleeping are closely linked.

Sleeping Aids

Can you encourage a child to use something to help him to get to sleep? I have heard that some parents put a special toy in the cot from birth, in the hope the baby will associate this toy with getting to sleep. My health visitor has suggested I get my child to start liking a blanket or a sheet, or a teddy, so this can be produced in moments when it's hard for her to get to sleep.
I have known many children who have always slept with a favourite 'thing' of one sort or another. They cry if they don't have it, and are instantly peaceful when it's produced. It stays with them at night, and sometimes in the day, as a comforter. These objects become an important part of family life – where the family goes, the blanket/teddy/doll/cloth goes too. Sensible parents spot the attachment growing and get a spare in (or a few spares if possible) for the time when it's in the

wash or (horrors) actually lost or left behind somewhere. If the favourite thing is a cloth or sheet or similar, you can cut it up without your child objecting – it's often just a corner they need to feel or suck, anyway. One little girl I knew was happy with a few scraps at a time of her special scarf.

It's interesting to note that the Americans call these objects 'lovies', and the child does seem to develop a loving, passionate attachment to them. They're also known as transitional objects, in psycho-speak, as they are reckoned to bridge the gap between mother and child.

I don't know whether you can be sure of actually engineering this need as a way of always having something to hand to encourage sleep ... but it's worth a try. My guess is that if a child needs this sort of help, and will benefit from it, she will find it in whatever there is to hand. But there can be no harm in making it easier for her to find something. Try it, if you like.

Checking Didn't Work ...

My daughter is 21 months old, and after never having an unbroken night since she was born we decided to do something positive. Maybe we should have done something sooner, but to be honest, after she was about six months things were much better than they had been before and we were too scared of rocking the boat and making her wake more often.

But the situation didn't continue its improvement, and in the last couple of months two things have happened – I have found out I am pregnant again, and she has started waking up twice instead of once. She has also started to be difficult to get into bed in the first place. I really couldn't face the prospect of having two wakeful children and I knew I want the whole thing sorted before this next baby is born. So we tried the 'checking' method. The first night we went in every two or three minutes and this lasted for three and a half hours before she settled. The second night was just the same – and the third night we decided we couldn't leave her to cry again and we abandoned it. Did we do something wrong or is this a method that just won't work for our daughter?

Questions

It could be that now just isn't the right time to change your daughter's sleeping pattern. You may feel under pressure to get the whole thing right, as if there's a deadline – which I suppose there is, seeing that you want things sorted out before the new baby comes, but presumably that is a good few months away.

I would suggest you leave things as they are for another couple of weeks before thinking again. It may be that your daughter needs to learn about settling down for the night first, without being expected to sleep through as well. Try and establish a routine for bedtime, at a time you feel is reasonable (if you have no idea, consider aiming for an 8 o'clock bedtime at first, and then making it sooner over a period of a few nights). Once you have this under your belt, as it were, think about doing the checking method again. This time, leave it a bit longer than two to three minutes before going in; make sure you are calm and quiet and boring ... don't let her think she has a chance of getting up and playing.

It may help you to have support from other parents, or from your health visitor. Tell her your situation, and ask for her advice.

Hyperactive?

I've been told my son is probably hyperactive because he is on the go the whole day – and most of the night. He is almost three and he has never shown any sign of sleeping through the night or of going to bed without a fuss. He does go to sleep sometimes, perhaps when we are out in the car or if he's sitting watching TV. I have tried cutting out foods with additives in them and stopping him from drinking orange squash, but it doesn't make any difference. He is very hard to control and I know they have problems with him at his nursery. I really am at my wit's end with him, as anything I say makes no difference to him at all.

Please get help. Some children do have real behavioural difficulties as well as giving their parents broken nights. Families like this need more help than a casual 'diagnosis' of hyperactivity. There are many parents who feel a change of diet to exclude certain foods has helped their children, and there has been research linking some foods (not necessarily foods with additives in – some ordinary foods cause reactions as well) with migraines and other aches and pains.

Do talk over your situation with someone who won't just dismiss your concerns. It may be that changing the way your son behaves generally will have a beneficial effect on his sleep, and that giving you good support will strengthen your ability to deal with him.

See your health visitor, your doctor, or your local child guidance unit (many take self-referrals). Your son's nursery teacher may also be able to refer you for help.

Cot to Bed?

What's the right age for a baby to move into a bed from a cot? My son is 18 months old, and we will need his cot for our new baby who is due in a couple of months. Would he be able to cope with a bed at this age? I'm still reluctant, as I can envisage him getting out and climbing downstairs or wandering around.

I think you're right to wonder about the impact of putting the new baby in what your son no doubt sees as 'his' cot. At 18 months it's hard enough to understand why a new little person has come into your life out of the blue without feeling your own special sleeping place has been nicked, too. But your new baby will be fine in a crib or cradle, a carry cot or pram top for at least three months or so – which gives you a little more time to play with.

Can your son stand up by himself in his cot? If so, chances are he'll soon be able to climb out, anyway, so that will stop being an issue. You may feel it's safer for him to climb out of a bed than out of a cot (with its risk of a bigger drop). A bed guard can prevent a fall from a bed.

Think about moving your son into a bed in the next couple of months. This will give him time to forget the cot was ever his own by the time your new baby needs it. Make the new bed his own by putting his usual and favourite cot toys in it or near it, and make a huge deal of saying what a clever, big boy he is, with his own big boy's bed.

The issue of getting out of bed and wandering can be dealt with by putting a safety gate across the doorway to his room, if you worry he could fall down the stairs during his meanderings. If this isn't your main worry and you're just concerned he will use his new-found mobility to be a bit of a nuisance and spoil your evenings you may have to be firm. Every time he comes to you, take him back without comment. Do it often enough, and stay consistent, and you will find he gets sick of bothering. The key is consistency: if sometimes he gets a cuddle, a biscuit and a story, you can't blame him for trying it on. Tell any babysitters to follow your policy, as well.

Sleeping and Working

I went back to work six months ago when my daughter Hannah was 12 months old. I collect her from the childminder at about 6 p.m., and she almost always falls asleep in the back of the car on the way home. That recharges her batteries, I'm afraid, and she is just not ready to go to bed for the night until 9.30 or 10 p.m. Is there any way round this situation?

Hannah probably needs that early evening sleep. It would be very difficult – and unsafe – to try to keep her awake while driving, though I expect you've already tried the safe and easy options like singing and talking loudly.

I'd suggest you get together with your childminder and work out a strategy to cope. It may be that your minder can encourage Hannah to have an afternoon nap at about 3.30 or 4. This might mean a bit of re-jigging if Hannah is used to sleeping straight after lunch, for example, but if your childminder is consistent – waking Hannah up if she does fall asleep at midday, for example – she should find that she can change Hannah's pattern after a few weeks at most.

Back to Work

I am about to go back to work part-time in four weeks, when my son Joe will be six months old. My mother will look after him on the two days I am at work. My problem is that he only ever falls asleep on the breast, day or night. I am dreading leaving him knowing he just won't be able to sleep without me.

My guess is that you will discover you don't actually need to worry quite so much. It may help to reassure you if you leave Joe with your mum for a 'dry run' before you actually go back to work. She may develop her own skills in helping him sleep, or he may just drop off without any real effort on anyone else's part. You won't be around, and Joe won't actually 'expect' a breastfeed because of this. If he feels secure and cared for, and he has a full tummy, he is likely to adapt to this change in his sleeping habits.

Useful Addresses

National Childbirth Trust
Alexandra House
Oldham Terrace
London W3 6NH
Tel: 0181–992 8637

Support for parents before and after birth. Antenatal classes; breastfeeding counselling.

CRY-SIS
BM Cry-sis
London WC1N 3XX
Tel: 0171–404 5011

Support for parents of crying babies.

Child Psychotherapy Trust
c/o Tavistock Centre
Belsize Lane
London NW3 5BA
Tel: 0171–435 7111

Index

babies:
    newborn 1, 8–20
    older 21–33
bed sharing 37, 39, 45–8, 76
bottle feeding 12–13, 32, 85
breastfeeding 6, 13–15, 32, 60, 81–2, 86

checking 40, 48, 88
colic 8, 18–19, 33
cot to bed 90
cot death 45, 46, 81
cranial osteopathy 68, 72
crying 9, 10–11, 19, 41–5, 74

daytime sleep 16
doctor 62
drugs 67–8
dummies 30, 79

early waking 26–8, 83

family bed *see* bed sharing
fears at bedtime 55–6, 77

health visitors 61–2
hospital 66–7, 74
hyperactivity 89

massage 10

naps 1, 24, 25–6
nightmares 33, 52, 54
night:
    terrors 57–8
    waking 28–33, 36, 60, 72

post-natal depression 80
psychotherapy 68–9

rituals 49, 50
routines 22-6

settling problems 2, 15, 49, 71
sleep clinics 62–5, 75
sleeping:
    aids 87
    position 80–81
spoiling 17

teething 32
toddlers 6, 34–51